SHIPWRECKS OF T.

SHIPWRECKS
OF THE
FORTH

INCLUDING WRECKS FROM
BERWICK ON TWEED TO STONEHAVEN

BOB BAIRD

NEKTON BOOKS
1993

Although reasonable care has been taken in preparing this book, the Publishers and Author respectively accept no responsibility or liability for any errors, omissions or alterations, or for any consequences ensuing upon the use of, or reliance upon, any information contained herein. Due caution should be exercised by anyone attempting dives on any wreck herein described or indicated. The Author and Publishers would be glad to hear of any inaccuracies or any new relevant material.

SHIPWRECKS OF THE FORTH
BY BOB BAIRD

ISBN 1 897995 00 8 Paper bound edition
ISBN 1 897995 01 6 Hard back edition

Copyright © Nekton Books 1993

All rights reserved. No part of this publication may be reproduced, stored in a retrieval system, or transmitted in any form or by any means, electronic, mechanical, photocopying, recording or otherwise , without the prior permission of the Publishers.

Published by Nekton Books,
94 Brownside Road, Cambuslang, Glasgow, G72 8AG
Telephone 041 641 4200.

Printed by Rannoch Press, Bearsden, Glasgow.

Cover design and internal layout grid by Ian Johnston
Maps and drawings by Bob Baird and Gordon Ridley
Halftones by John Stewart of Cordfall Ltd., Glasgow

Cover illustration: The wreck of the *Switha* on Herwit Rock (photograph by Bob Baird). Upper inset: HMS *Campania* sinking off Burntisland (photograph courtesy of Conway Picture Library)
Lower inset: Submarine *K-16*, sister vessel of the submarines *K-4* and *K-17* lost near the Isle of May (photograph courtesy of Ian Johnston).

All reasonable care has been taken to trace the owners of copyright pictures. Where it has not been possible to trace copyright, the publishers will meet any reasonable request if contacted by the owners of such copyright.

The database upon which this book is based was prepared using Ashton Tate *dBase III+* running on an Amstrad *PC1640* computer. This was coverted into *WordStar* files and ported into Macintosh format in Microsoft *Word 5.1* using *Apple File Exchange*. These files were imported in Aldus *PageMake 4.2* running on an Apple Macintosh *Quadra 700* computer, along with illustrations produced using Adobe *Illustrator 3.2* and photographs that were image processed within Adobe *Photoshop 2.0.1*. The text is set in *Goudy* 10 point.

Contents

Page

Chapter 1 : Introduction — 10

Chapter 2 : Berwick, Eyemouth, St. Abbs & Dunbar — 20

Chapter 3 : North Berwick, Aberlady & Leith — 48

Chapter 4 : Inchkeith, Inchcolm & Rosyth — 68

Chapter 5 : Kirkcaldy, Methil & Elie — 98

Chapter 6 : Isle of May — 112

Chapter 7 : Fife Ness — 146

Chapter 8 : Tay & Arbroath — 164

Chapter 9 : Montrose, Gourdon & Stonehaven — 180

Chapter 10 : Unknown wrecks — 198

Appendix 1 : Analysis of losses — 200

Appendix 2 : Diving information — 201

Appendix 3 : Bibliography — 202

Index of wrecks by name — 203

Index of wrecks by latitude — 209

Photographs

	Page
X-craft in Aberlady Bay	61
Switha (stern view)	70
Switha (starboard view)	71
Campania as a liner	81
Campania as an aircraft carrier	81
Campania sinking before dawn	82
Campania sinking 8.00 am	82
Campania sinking 8.20 am	82
Campania sinking 8.30 am	83
Campania sinking 8.40 am	83
Campania resting on seabed	83
Salvestria in harbour	88
Royal Archer underway	100
The remains of the *Thomas L. Devlin*	133
K-4 aground on Walney Island	140
K-16, sister vessel of *K-4* and *K-17*	141
K-6 (without bulbous bow)	141
Clan Shaw docked	169
HMS *Argyll* at speed	175
Reindeer underway	194
Granero aground	195

Maps & Diagrams

	Page
Map of Scotland showing area covered herein	8
Map of South east Scotland showing chapter areas	9
Table of the points and quarter points of the compass	16
Diagram of the points and quarter points of the compass	17
Diagram of the Single Oropesa Sweep	18
Diagram of the drift or bar sweep	19
Map of the wrecks lying off Berwick, Eyemouth & St. Abbs	21
Location map of the *President*	24
Location map of the *Alfred Erlandsen*	26
Location map of the *Odense*	28
Location map and transits for the *Glanmire*	30
Map of the wrecks lying off Dunbar	33
Map of the wrecks lying off North Berwick & Aberlady	49
Location map and transit for HMS *Ludlow*	52
Sketch of the *Royal Fusilier* on the seabed	55
Location map and transits for the *Royal Fusilier*	56
Location map and transits for the *Chester II*	64
Map of the wrecks lying off the island of Inchkeith	69
Location map and transits for the *Runswick*	73
Location map and transits for the *Sappho*	75
Location map for the *Campania*	84
Location map and transits for the *Salvestria*	89
Map of the wrecks lying off Kirkcaldy, Methil & Elie	99
Map of the wrecks lying off the Isle of May	113
Map of the wrecks near the Isle of May	123
The locations of the *Island* and the *Anlaby*	126
The locations of the *Thomas L. Devlin* and the *Mars*	134
Map of the location of the *Battle of May Isle*	143
Diagram showing the progress of the *Battle of May Isle*	144
Map of the wrecks around Fife Ness	147
Location map of the *Chingford*	152
Map of the wrecks lying off the Tay estuary	165
Map of the wrecks between Arbroath and Montrose	181
Map of the wrecks between Gourdon and Stonehaven	189

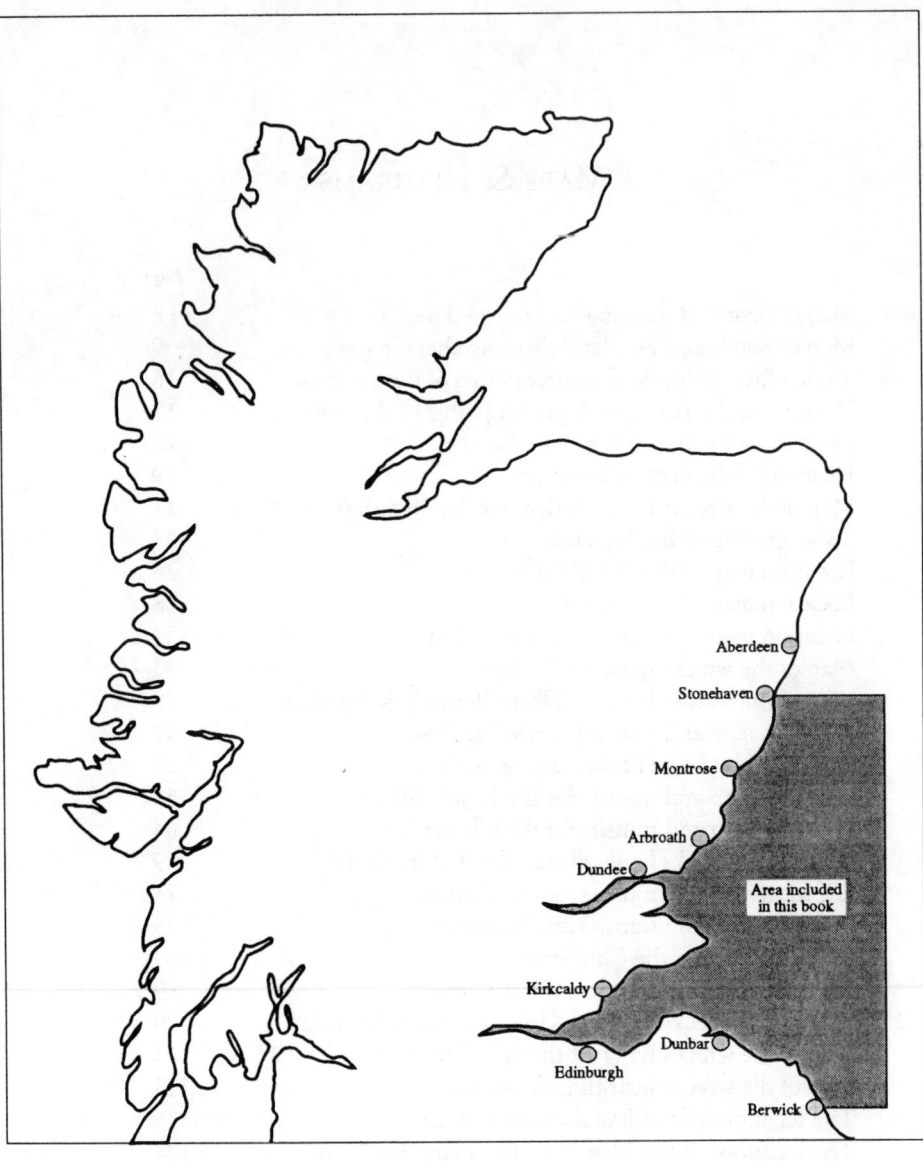

Map of Scotland showing the area covered by this book

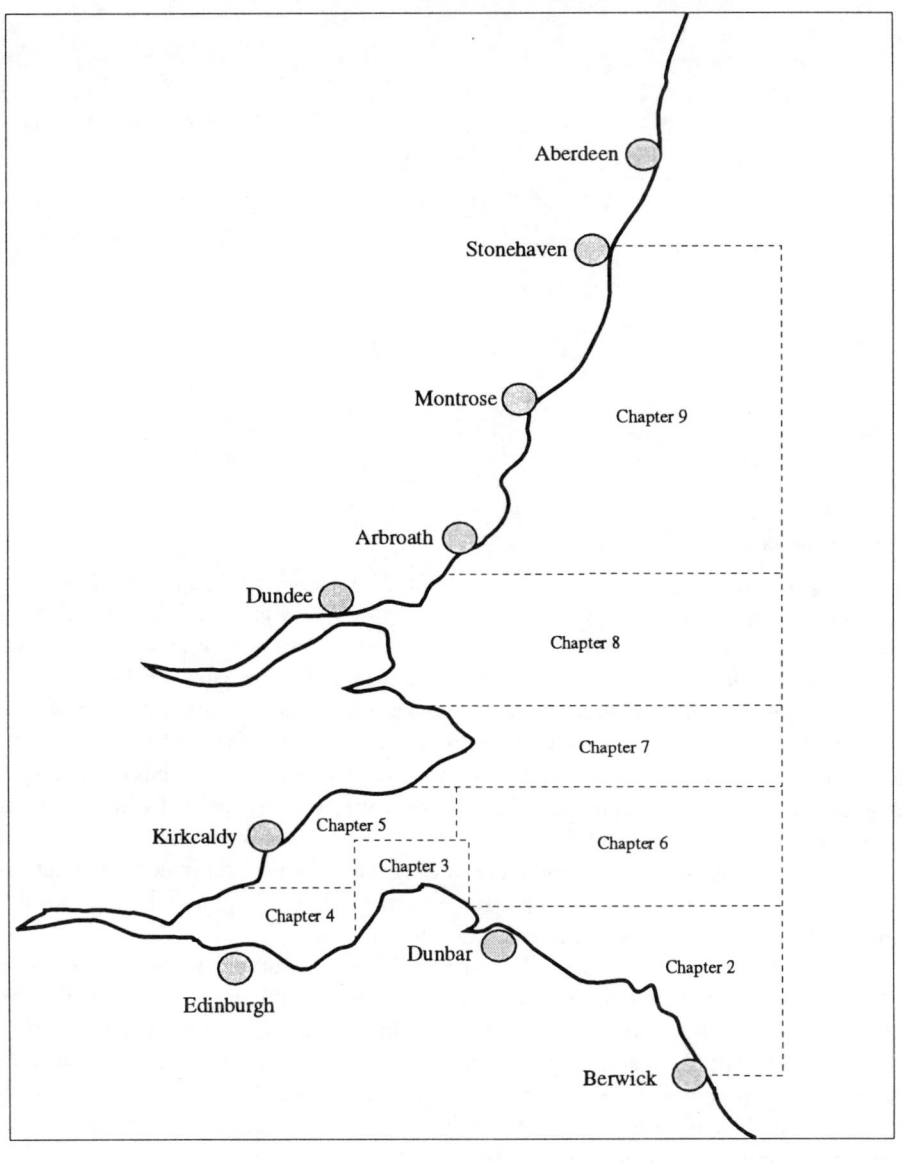

Map of part of East Scotland showing the area covered by each chapter

CHAPTER 1

INTRODUCTION

FIRST WORDS

For as long as I can remember I have been fascinated by ships, wrecks, and marine salvage, and over the years, have read many books and articles, and gathered diverse pieces of information on this subject. Since taking up diving as a hobby some 13 years ago, my interest has been further developed and focused mainly on wrecks in Scottish waters.

The information I had collected over the years was in a chaotic state until I transferred it on to a computer system, starting with wrecks of the Forth. The facility for cross-relating standardised data enabled snippets of information from various sources to be compared and assessed, and an orderly picture began to emerge. I very quickly realised I had the basic details for a book on the subject, and all that was required to make it more than merely a list, was some further research to add meat to the bones, both for the sheer enjoyment of extending my own personal knowledge, and also to make it a more useful and enjoyable source of information to those with a similar interest.

Others had already written carefully researched books about shipwrecks in the Clyde, and elsewhere in Britain, but no-one had written a book about shipwrecks in the Forth. This book was originally intended to be just that, but in my quest for further information on wrecks in the Forth, I kept stumbling on references to wrecks in other areas, and with the discovery of each new piece of information, the area covered by my data base gradually expanded to include the entire East coast of Scotland, the North coast, and the West coast from Cape Wrath down to Sanda Island off the Mull of Kintyre.

Most divers are keen to dive on wrecks and to learn something about them, although there is some reluctance amongst divers to divulge jealously-guarded wreck information to other divers, who often tend to be regarded as potential competitors. I have found from personal experience, however, that being willing to share my knowledge with others generally brings its own rewards in the form of reciprocal information and friendships with fellow enthusiasts, and has vastly improved the quality of my own diving.

THIS BOOK

Research for a book of this nature can never be wholly complete, but one has to stop at some point to produce the first edition. This book contains details of a representative selection of over 300 Forth wrecks from my data base which at the present time includes at least another 500 in that area alone. Further information will inevitably come to my attention aided, I hope, by input from others, including readers of this book. Perhaps at some future date, if a sufficiently large amount of new information is forthcoming to justify it, an updated second edition may eventually be produced.

Many of the wrecks in this book are not charted, but all charted wrecks in the area have been included, and while this book has been written primarily for the interest of fellow divers, some of the wrecks are too deep for sport diving, and are therefore likely to be only of academic interest to divers. The locations of the deeper wrecks may be of more practical interest to fishermen, however, as it is well known that wrecks attract fish, and some of the wrecks are popular with sea anglers.

To add to my own knowledge, I should be grateful for any further information which readers may be able to provide. Knowing a date for the sinking of a vessel provides a good starting point for personal research through the files of local newspapers, unless the date is during the first or second world wars, when censorship prevented newspapers from publishing information which would now be useful to wreck detectives.

Some of the named wrecks whose positions are not accurately known will no doubt tie up with some of the charted wrecks which have yet to be identified. Others will be the remains of vessels for which, through lack of sufficient information, I am presently unable to suggest a possible name with any degree of confidence. Naturally, I would be willing to attempt to identify any wreck found which does not appear to be included in this book.

As I have personally dived on only a tiny proportion of these wrecks, (and as far as I am aware, the vast majority are completely undived), I should welcome further details from divers visiting any of the wrecks, to let me know what was found, possibly enabling identification of an *Unknown*, or to correct any errors of fact or omission I may have made.

WRECK RESEARCH

The information in this book has been gleaned over a number of years from many sources, including newspaper files, the Admiralty Hydrographic Department, and Lloyds. In addition, many books and other publications have provided useful information, as, indeed have many individuals. Wartime losses are particularly difficult to research because the strict censorship which applied during these periods suppressed information from the public domain. As a result, wartime newspapers are not very helpful. The Patrick Stephens reprint of the HMSO publication *British Vessels Lost at Sea 1914-1918 and 1939-1945* was one of the principal sources of information on wartime losses of British ships, but when referring to that source, be aware that the positions given are generally estimates of the position at the time of attack. No doubt in some instances the vessel sank almost immediately, but in others, the actual sinking may not have occurred for some considerable time after the attack, (up to several days later in some cases), during which period the damaged vessel may still have been under power, or taken in tow before sinking, or merely drifted for a time before finally foundering or being driven ashore.

It has long been a matter of regret to me that the dates of first reporting of charted wrecks are not given on the charts, as that would be a considerable aid to identifying them, or at the very least, eliminating some of the speculation regarding their possible identities. For example, a wreck first reported in 1920 is extremely unlikely to be a ship known to have sunk in 1940! For some wrecks several slightly different positions have been recorded over the years, and I have generally accepted information dated 1987, for example, as being more accurate than a 1919 position for the same wreck. This is not because the wreck has moved in the intervening period, but simply reflects the greater accuracy resulting from continuing advances in electronic navigation technology.

It used to be said that if you asked a young merchant navy officer where his ship was, he would confidently make a precise dot on the chart with a sharp pencil. A more experienced officer would draw a circle around the dot, and the older and wiser the officer, the larger the circle would be. With his years of experience in navigating across the oceans, the Captain would probably describe a fairly large circle on the chart with his finger and say "Somewhere in this area".

I have done my best to select what I consider to be perhaps the most accurate of the sometimes vague and conflicting information available. When an exact position is not known, I have endeavoured to provide as close an estimate as the information currently available to me will permit, and this is indicated in the text.

THE WRECK DETAILS

The wrecks are described from South to North (i.e. in latitude order) and in an approximately clockwise direction within the Firth of Forth.

Detailed information on each wreck is given immediately under the vessel's name. This is followed by details of the circumstances of the loss of the vessel, its present wherabouts and condition (where known) and other more general information where this is known.

Any vessel can be found by reference to the two indexes - a name index and a latitude index. These give both the page number and the wreck number (these are assigned sequentially throughout the book).

MAPS AND CHARTS

For maximum comprehension of, and benefit from, the information provided in this book, it is recommended that it should be read in conjunction with the following Admiralty charts:

        Chart No. 175 - Fife Ness to St.Abbs Head.
        Chart No. 734 - Isle of May to Inchkeith.
        Chart No. 735 - North Craig to Oxcars.
        Chart No. 736 - Oxcars to Rosyth.
        Chart No. 737 - Rosyth to Grangemouth.

―――――――――――――――― INTRODUCTION ――――――――――――――――

The Ordnance Survey 1:50,000 Landranger series maps, (sheets 59, 65, 66, 67 and 75), would also provide a useful reference guide while reading this book, particularly in respect of the many vessels which were lost through running aground.

The 1:25000 Ordnance Survey Pathfinder are also most useful. The coastline of the Forth is covered in some 11 sheets, with a further 10 covering the outlying coasts.

FORTH SHIPPING AND SHIPWRECKS

The Forth has been one of several important Scottish shipping areas for many centuries. The early coastal trade was not as prolific as that of the West Coast, but it was still important in its day. Trade with Scandinavia has always featured in Forth shipping, in particular much of the Baltic wood trade came to Bo'ness and other Forth ports. The movement of coal by sea was central to early British trade and industry. Many ships also traded with the British Empire, the export of whisky being especially important. There has also been large amounts of naval shipping using the Forth for many years.

For much of the maritime history of the Forth, there were no lights or lighthouses and, furthermore, ships were at the mercy of the wind. The plethora of modern electronic navigation aids were a thing of the distant future. Many fine ships were lost to the above trades due to these circumstances. For instance, some 500 were lost between 1850 and 1900 alone. Earlier records are incomplete and elusive and obviously many more vessels must have been lost.

More recently, by far the most common causes of shipwrecks are running aground and collisions, while during both wars, submarine torpedoes, mines, and attack by aircraft were additional hazards which accounted for a substantial number of the wrecks.

A HISTORICAL COINCIDENCE

The Forth has the unenviable distinction of having been the scene of both the first and the last enemy attacks on the British mainland during the Second World War.

The first German aircraft to be shot down over the UK in the Second World War were two *Ju*-88s on a bombing raid on ships anchored off Rosyth dockyard, shot down by *Spitfires* piloted by Flt. Lt. Pat Gifford of 603 (City of Edinburgh) Sqdn. and Flt. Lt. George Pinkerton of 602 (City of Glasgow) Squadron on 16th October 1939. One fell into the sea about 4 miles NE of Port Seton at 14.55 hrs., the other 3 miles east of Crail. Helmut Pohle, the pilot of that *Ju*-88, and George Pinkerton, who shot him down, have never met, but both are farmers, and have been engaged in friendly correspondence with each other for many years. The *Ju*-88 off Port Seton was raised about two weeks later, and taken to Leith, but as far as I know the other was never recovered, and the remains will still be there.

Off the Isle of May lie the wrecks of the last British and Norwegian ships to be sunk during WW2, both, sadly, with loss of life, in the very last hour of the War. (These were the *Avondale Park*, wreck No.162, and the *Sneland I*, wreck No. 165, respectively.)

LIMITATIONS OF THE FORTH FOR WRECK DIVERS

By far the greatest concentration of wreck diving activity around mainland Scotland is in the Clyde, and I am convinced that relatively few are aware that South East Scotland and the Forth has hundreds of wrecks to offer, ranging from an aircraft carrier to midget submarines, and almost everything in between, most of them totally undived!

There are several reasons for this.
- Many of the Forth wrecks are in a very much wider part of the river than is the case with the most popular wrecks in the Clyde, and its waters are much more exposed to wind and weather from all directions, but especially to any wind with an easterly component.
- A significant number of the wrecks are there because others, including very experienced seamen, have underestimated the effect of the weather on the waters of the Forth.
- When there is no wind, very often low-lying fog, mist or haze causes many of the wreck positions to be completely out of sight of land, making location by the normal use of transits impossible.
- Even on a good day, the distances from land are often too great to enable small details such as individual buildings to be distinguished sufficiently well to provide useful transits in conjunction with more readily identifiable features such as islands, hills, power station chimneys, radio masts or the massive Forth bridges. These larger features are of remarkably limited use for obtaining wreck transits, as it is hard to find anything else visible to line up with them! The formula for calculating the distance in nautical miles to the radar horizon is the square root of the height of the scanner (in feet) multiplied by 1.22. The eyes of someone sitting in an inflatable boat are likely to be no more than about 4 ft. above the water surface, in which case the horizon is 2.44 nautical miles away. Even standing up, eye level will be only about 6 ft. above the water surface, and the horizon will be 2.99 nautical miles away. This means that the shore line beyond that distance is not visible, as, due to the curvature of the Earth, it will be beyond and below the horizon. Hence, objects on the shore line can not be seen from distances beyond the horizon. Only the tops of objects such as hills which stick up over the horizon will be visible, but not their bases.
- Anyone who has tried to position a small boat accurately over a wreck, using only hand-held compass bearings to points a long distance across open water, will know the degree of inaccuracy inherent in that method of position fixing!

DIVING THE FORTH WRECKS

As a result, diving the wrecks in the Forth tends to be a much more difficult proposition altogether than diving those in the Clyde. Apart from seaworthy boats, echo sounders and accurate navigation and position fixing equipment such as Decca are absolutely essential for finding a great many of the wrecks. A magnetometer would also be of considerable assistance, but it is only in recent years that these electronic aids have become relatively common items of equipment for many divers. Availability of this equipment does not in itself, however, provide the complete answer to all of the problems. It is still necessary to know where to look for the wrecks, and that information is provided, to the best of my

Introduction

ability, in this book. To compensate for the lack of available transits for the majority of the wrecks, I have endeavoured to give Decca positions.

Hiring a local trawler is probably still the best practical solution for many divers who wish to explore those wrecks located a long way offshore. This has the additional advantage of the skipper's local knowledge and experience, along with all the technological equipment and comfort provided by a relatively large vessel.

Access to the water for boats leaves a lot to be desired. There are remarkably few launching slip facilities provided on the shores of the Forth, and those that do exist are tidal. The harbours from which the fishing boats operate are also tidal, affecting the potential times of departure and return. Surface conditions can vary enormously throughout the Forth, from flat calm with clear visibility at one point, while simultaneously, there may be heaving seas and severely curtailed visibility at another. At some places, tidal streams and currents run far more strongly than the charts suggest, making slack water and first class boat handling more than ordinarily important.

Underwater visibility also varies considerably from one part of the Forth to another. It is normally excellent from Inchkeith seawards, where most of the wrecks lie, while upriver of Inchkeith, visibility deteriorates rapidly to virtually zero from Inchcolm westwards.

Acknowledgements

I am indebted to a number of individuals who have provided useful information, and would especially like to thank Gordon Ridley and Ian Whittaker for their invaluable assistance with information, encouragement and technological support in this book's preparation.

Note

Some of the wrecks listed in this book may be considered to be War Graves - notably K-4 and HMS Pathfinder.

War Graves are covered by the Protection of Military Remains Act 1986 *and include the wrecks of any Royal Navy ship or merchant vessel lost on active Government service and which have human remains aboard.*

Apparently it is normally permissible to dive on these wrecks but not to disturb or remove anything from the site.

PLEASE RESPECT THESE FACTS

The Compass

Modern compasses have a scale marked in degrees, with 0 at North round clockwise to 360 again at North. In days gone by, the compass rose was marked in *Points* and *Quarter Points*. Some compass cards are marked with both degrees and points, the degrees being on the outside. There are 32 compass points in a circle of 360 degrees. One point, therefore, equals 11.25 degrees, and a quarter point, which is the smallest division shown on a card marked in that way, equals marginally under 3 degrees. (2.8125 degrees). The illustration opposite shows the compass and the names of the points and quarter points and the table below gives their equivalence in degrees. Note that none of the by-points or quarter points takes its name from a three-letter point: For example, N by E is correct, not NNE by N, and NE by $N^3/_4N$ is correct, not $NNE^1/_4E$.

Point	Heading	Point	Heading	Point	Heading	Point	Heading
NORTH	0	EAST	90	SOUTH	180	WEST	270
N 1/4 E	2.8125	E 1/4 S	92.8125	S 1/4 W	182.8125	W 1/4 N	272.8125
N 1/2 E	5.625	E 1/2 S	95.625	S 1/2 W	185.625	W 1/2 N	275.625
N 3/4 E	8.4375	E 3/4 S	98.4375	S 3/4 W	188.4375	W 3/4 N	278.4375
N by E	11.25	E by S	101.25	S by W	191.25	W by N	281.25
N by E 1/4 E	14.0625	E by S 1/4 S	104.0625	S by W 1/4 W	194.0625	W by N 1/4 N	284.0625
N by E 1/2 E	16.875	E by S 1/2 S	106.875	S by W 1/2 W	196.875	W by N 1/2 N	286.875
N by E 3/4 E	19.6875	E by S 3/4 S	109.6875	S by W 3/4 W	199.6875	W by N 3/4 N	289.6875
NNE	22.5	ESE	112.5	SSW	202.5	WNW	292.5
NE by N 3/4 N	25.3125	SE by E 3/4 E	115.3125	SW by W 3/4 S	205.3125	NW by W 3/4 W	295.3125
NE by N 1/2 N	28.125	SE by E 1/2 E	118.125	SW by W 1/2 S	208.125	NW by W 1/2 W	298.125
NE by N 1/4 N	30.9375	SE by E 1/4 E	120.9375	SW by W 1/4 S	210.9375	NW by W 1/4 W	300.9375
NE by N	33.75	SE by E	123.75	SW by W	213.75	NW by W	303.75
NE 3/4 E	36.5625	SE 3/4 E	126.5625	SW 3/4 W	216.5625	NW 3/4 W	306.5625
NE 1/2 N	39.375	SE 1/2 E	129.375	SW 1/2 W	219.375	NW 1/2 W	309.375
NE 1/4 N	42.1875	SE 1/4 E	132.1875	SW 1/4 W	222.1875	NW 1/4 W	312.1875
NORTH EAST	45	SOUTH EAST	135	SOUTH WEST	225	NORTH WEST	315
NE 1/4 E	47.8125	SE 1/4 S	137.8125	SW 1/4 W	227.8125	NW 1/4 N	317.8125
NE 1/2 E	50.625	SE 1/2 S	140.625	SW 1/2 W	230.625	NW 1/2 N	320.625
NE 3/4 E	53.4375	SE 3/4 S	143.4375	SW 3/4 W	233.4375	NW 3/4 N	323.4375
NE by E	56.25	SE by S	146.25	SW by W	236.25	NW by N	326.25
NE by E 1/4 E	59.0625	SE by S 1/4 S	149.0625	SW by W 1/4 W	239.0625	NW by N 1/4 W	329.0625
NE by E 1/2 E	61.875	SE by S 1/2 S	151.875	SW by W 1/2 W	241.875	NW by N 1/2 W	331.875
NE by E 3/4 E	64.6875	SE by S 3/4 S	154.6875	SW by W 3/4 W	244.6875	NW by N 3/4 W	334.6875
ENE	67.5	SSE	157.5	WSW	247.5	NNW	337.5
E by N 3/4 N	70.3125	S by E 3/4 E	160.3125	W by S 3/4 S	250.3125	N by W 1/4 N	340.3125
E by N 1/2 N	73.125	S by E 1/2 E	163.125	W by S 1/2 S	253.125	N by W 1/2 N	343.125
E by N 1/4 N	75.9375	S by E 1/4 E	165.9375	W by S 1/4 S	255.9375	N by W 3/4 N	345.9375
E by N	78.75	S by E	168.75	W by S	258.75	N by W	348.75
E 3/4 N	81.5625	S 3/4 E	171.5625	W 3/4 S	261.5625	N 3/4 W	351.5625
E 1/2 N	84.375	S 1/2 E	174.375	W 1/2 S	264.375	N 1/2 W	354.375
E 1/4 N	87.1875	S 1/4 E	177.1875	W 1/4 S	267.1875	N 1/4 W	357.1875
EAST	90	SOUTH	180	WEST	270	NORTH	360

INTRODUCTION

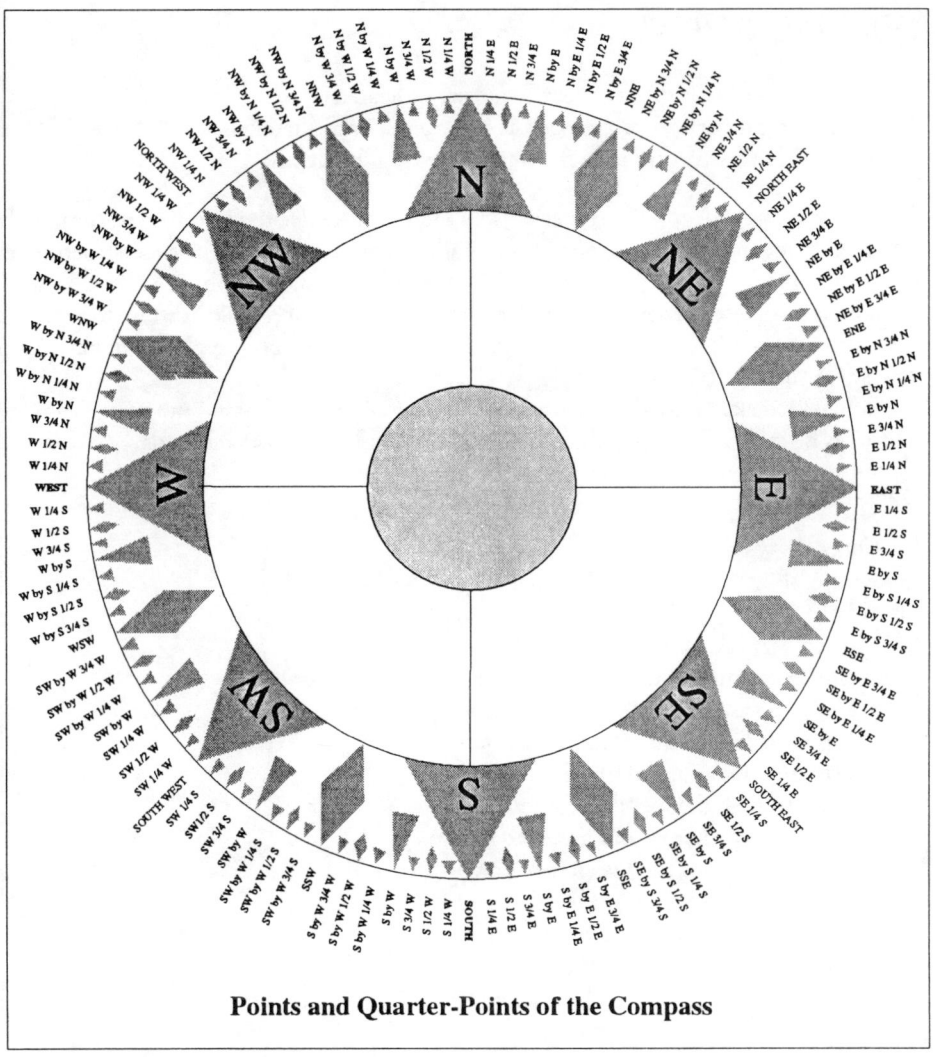

Points and Quarter-Points of the Compass

The present metric series of Admiralty charts have compass roses marked in degrees true, on the outside of the rose, and degrees magnetic, on the inside, the difference between them being the local magnetic variation. The amount and direction of the annual change is also given within the compass rose.

If information concerning the position of a wreck includes a compass bearing, it is important to note the date from which the bearing originates, and to take account of the local magnetic variation in the area over the years which have elapsed since the date of the information.

SWEEPING OF WRECKS

Charted wrecks which have been swept are indicated on the chart by a bar with upright vertical projections at either end, immediately below the Wk symbol which contains a figure representing the depth.

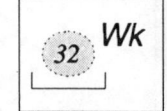

The word *swept*, as applied to wrecks, is commonly misunderstood, and often erroneously presumed to mean that a sweep wire has literally swept, or removed, the superstructure off a sunken vessel for the purpose of increasing the safe clearance depth.

This is complete nonsense. It would require a wire of infinite breaking strain to be towed by a ship of infinite power and propeller efficiency, and could only apply to wrecks which were sitting upright on the bottom.

When a wreck is said to have been swept, this simply means that its minimum clearance depth has been determined by the use of one of the following two methods:

OROPESA SWEEP

The Oropesa sweep used by mine sweepers was named after the ship in which it was first tried out in 1918.

A heavy torpedo-shaped float took the sweep wire out on to the mine sweeper's quarter, about 500 yards astern. An *otter* attached to the sweep wire below this float, and a *kite* attached to the wire immediately astern of the trawler, controlled the depth of the wire, working on the principle of air kites. The kite held the inboard end of the sweep wire down in the water, while the otter at the other end kept the sweep wire curving out about 250 yards on the mine sweeper's quarter.

The mine sweeper following behind steamed just inside the limit of the other's curving sweep, and in larger groups, every following vessel did the same, so that only the lead ship was at risk from mines as she nosed into unswept waters.

The serrated sweep wire cut the mooring cables of the mines, which were exploded or sunk by gunfire as they bobbed to the surface.

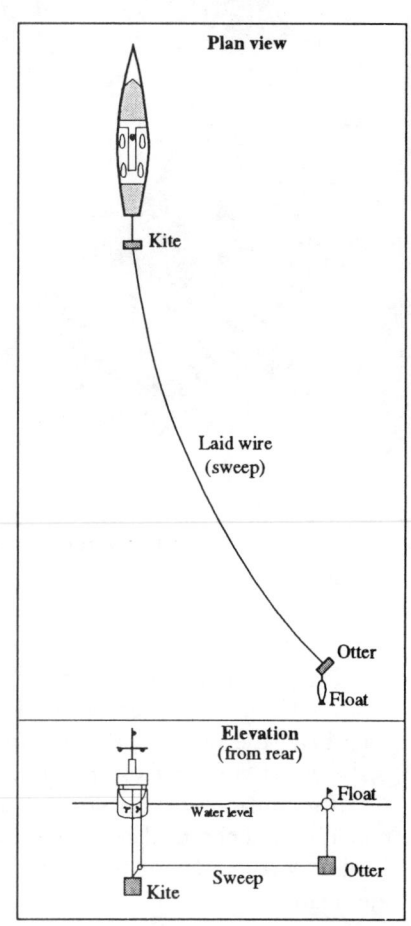

The Single Oropesa sweep

BAR OR DRIFT SWEEP

In this alternative, more accurate, method of measuring the minimum depth of a wreck, a rigid iron bar is suspended horizontally below a ship drifting over the wreck. The bar is hung over the side on three measured lines - one at each end, and one in the middle to avoid any bending effect on the bar. The depth of the bar is adjusted until the bar just avoids fouling the wreck as the ship drifts over it.

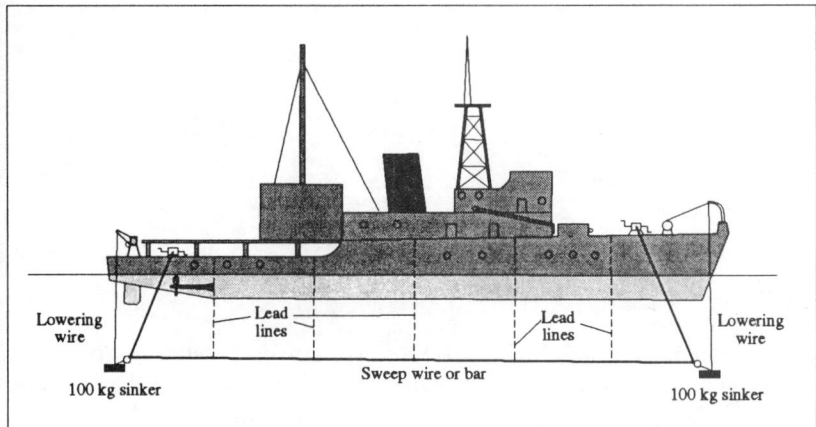

The bar or drift sweep

By computing the time of the measurement against tidal prediction tables, the depth is converted to chart datum.

Very often a heavy wire is used instead of a rigid bar. Note that the gear is put over the up-tide side of the vessel so that she will drift away with the tide from any snags.

TONNAGE

Gross tonnage: is a measure of space, not of weight, and indicates the total permanently enclosed space of a ship - i.e. her internal volume - and is calculated on the basis of 100 cubic feet. = 1 ton.

Net tonnage: is the Gross Tonnage less the space occupied by engines, boilers, bunkers, crew's quarters and all other space which, although essential for the working of the ship, is "non-earning". The Net Tonnage, therefore, indicates how much revenue-earning space there is in the ship.

Tons displacement: is the actual weight of the ship in long tons (2240 lbs. avoirdupois), as determined by the equivalent weight of water displaced by the ship when afloat.

Tons deadweight: is the total weight of cargo, fuel, stores, crew and all other items which are not actually a part of the ship, but which the ship can carry when she is floating down to her load marks.

CHAPTER 2

THE WRECKS OF BERWICK, EYEMOUTH, ST. ABBS & DUNBAR

INTRODUCTION

This stretch of coast is almost entirely rocky and cliff-lined, with deep water close off shore. By contrast with the more industrialised areas lying further West, much of the coastline between Berwick and Dunbar is still almost in its original wild state.

Some of the coves are reminiscent of Cornwall and, in fact, the history of the area abounds with tales of smugglers and their illicit activities. For instance, there is a multitude of stories about Fast Castle. One concerns a secret passageway in the cliffs connecting the Castle, which stands above the high cliffs, to the sea below. The Castle also has rumours of treasure of gold coin that has stimulated the imaginations of many people over the years to search afresh from both the Castle itself and, indeed, from a supposed underwater entrance to seaward. All of these searches have so far come to nought.

Reefs sprawling for miles below the cliffs have attracted divers from all over Britain since the beginnings of the sport in the 1950s.

The area does not contain any major port and the main harbours are those of Eyemouth, St. Abbs and Dunbar which concentrate mainly on fishing activities. Boat-launching access to the sea is available at Eyemouth, St. Abbs, Pease Bay and Dunbar. It may also be possible to hire a trawler from Dunbar.

On the Black Friday of 14th October 1881, while the Eyemouth fishing fleet was at sea, a great storm blew up and 23 of the boats were overwhelmed by tremendous waves. Those that were left struggled back to seek refuge in the harbour, only to be dashed to pieces on the rocks near the harbour entrance, within view of the horrified watchers on the shore. By the time the storm abated, 129 fishermen from Eyemouth had been lost, along with 60 from the neighbouring communities.

One hundred years later, in 1981, the people of Eyemouth had a commemorative tapestry made, and this is the centrepiece of the town's museum, which itself is a memorial to the victims of the great storm.

Berwick, Eyemouth, St. Abbs & Dunbar

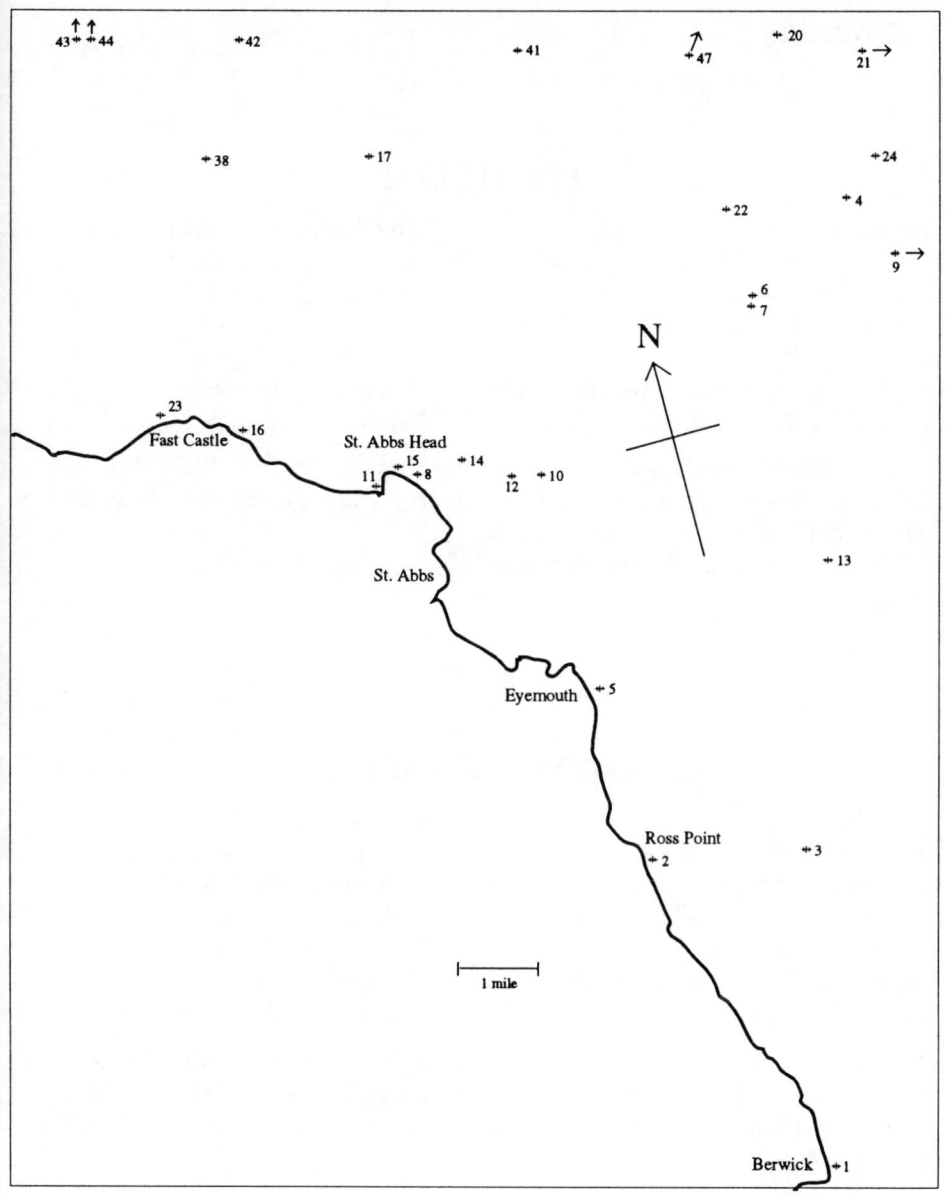

Chart showing the locations of the wrecks lying off the coast between Berwick and Fast Castle. Wrecks lying some distance offshore in the Firth of Forth are also shown.

The Wrecks

BEN HEILEM

Wreck No :	1	Date Sunk :	08 10 1917
Latitude :	55 46 01 N	Longitude :	01 59 00 W
Decca Lat :	5546.02 N	Decca Long :	0159.00 W
Location :	Just N of Berwick Harbour	Area :	Berwick
Type :	Trawler	Tonnage :	196 gross
Length :	115.1 feet Beam : 22.1 feet	Draught :	11.9 feet
How Sunk :	Ran aground	Depth :	metres

The 196 ton *Ben Heilem*, a steel screw ketch, (steam trawler), built in 1912 by Hall Russell of Aberdeen, was requisitioned for use as a mine sweeper during the first world war, and was armed with 12-pounder and 6-pounder guns.

She was wrecked just North of Berwick Harbour on 8th October 1917.

BARON STJERNBLAD

Wreck No :	2	Date Sunk :	23 04 1917
Latitude :	55 50 00 N PA	Longitude :	02 04 00 W PA
Decca Lat :	5550.00 N	Decca Long :	0204.00 W
Location :	SE of Ross Point, Burnmouth	Area :	Berwick
Type :	Steamship	Tonnage :	991 gross
Length :	203.9 feet Beam : 31.3 feet	Draught :	15.8 feet
How Sunk :	By submarine	Depth :	23 metres

The 991 ton Danish steel screw steamship *Baron Stjernblad*, built in 1890 by Motala M.V. of Gothenburg, was captured and sunk by a German submarine on 23rd April 1917.

She is now reported to lie in 23 metres of water close to the shore, South East of Ross Point near Berwick.

— BERWICK, EYEMOUTH, ST. ABBS & DUNBAR —

EGHOLM

Wreck No : 3	Date Sunk : 25 02 1945
Latitude : 55 50 00 N PA	Longitude : 01 52 00 W PA
Decca Lat : 5550.00 N	Decca Long : 0152.00 W
Location : Off Berwick	Area : Berwick
Type : Steamship	Tonnage : 1317 gross
Length : 254.6 feet Beam : 37.2 feet	Draught : 16.0 feet
How Sunk : Torpedoed by U-2322	Depth : metres

The 1317 ton British steamship *Egholm*, built in 1924, was torpedoed by *U-2322* (Heckel), off Berwick, in position 555000N, 015200W while en route from Leith to London. Two crew and three gunners were lost out of 23 crew and 3 gunners.

Peter Collings gives the depth of the wreck as 23 metres, but he also gives the position as 555500N, 015524W, which is 60 metres deep! If 23 metres is the correct depth, the position he gives cannot be correct.

There is a wreck charted at 555500N, 015600W, again in about 60 metres, very close to the position given by Mr. Collings, and this may be the *Egholm*.

MAGNE

Wreck No : 4	Date Sunk : 14 03 1945
Latitude : 55 51 12 N	Longitude : 01 55 24 W
Decca Lat : 5551.20 N	Decca Long : 0155.40 W
Location : Off Eyemouth	Area : Eyemouth
Type : Steamship	Tonnage : 1226 gross
Length : 246.9 feet Beam : 37.1 feet	Draught : 14.0 feet
How Sunk : Torpedoed by U-714	Depth : metres

While en route from Methil to London, the 1226 ton Swedish steamship *Magne* was torpedoed off Eyemouth by the *U-714* on 14th March 1945. Ten of her crew were lost. *U-714* was sunk later that same day by depth charges. There were no survivors.

PRESIDENT

Wreck No :	5	Date Sunk :	28 04 1928
Latitude :	55 52 05 N	Longitude :	02 04 15 W
Decca Lat :	5552.08 N	Decca Long :	0204.25 W
Location :	Whaltness, S of Eyemouth	Area :	Eyemouth
Type :	Steamship	Tonnage :	1945 gross
Length :	280.0 feet Beam : 40.5 feet	Draught :	18.2 feet
How Sunk :	Ran aground	Depth :	10 metres

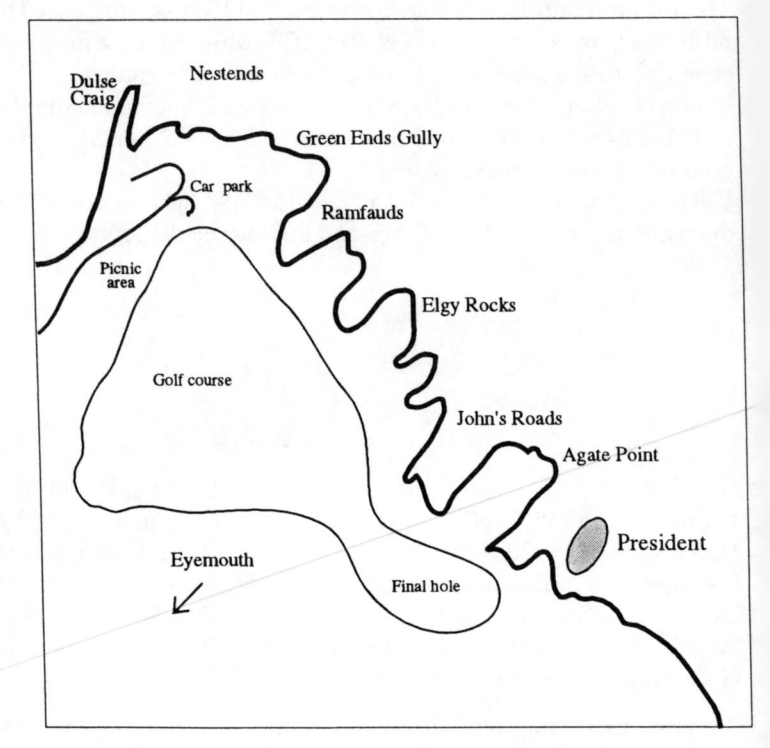

The location of the President off Whaltness, Eyemouth

The 1945 ton steamship *President*, built in 1907 by S.P. Austin & Son of Sunderland, ran ashore under the cliffs at Whaltness, 150 metres North of Scout Point, just South of Eyemouth, while en route from Hamburg to Methil. The crew were able to scramble ashore using a ladder!

The wreck is broken up in shallow water close inshore near Whalt Point, at the South corner of the golf course.

CRAMOND ISLAND

Wreck No :	6	Date Sunk :	02 04 1941
Latitude :	55 52 30 N	Longitude :	02 01 00 W
Decca Lat :	5552.50 N	Decca Long :	0201.00 W
Location :	120° 5 miles off St. Abbs Head	Area :	St. Abbs
Type :	Trawler	Tonnage :	180 gross
Length :	112.3 feet Beam : 21.9 feet	Draught :	11.3 feet
How Sunk :	By aircraft	Depth :	64 metres

At 14.04 hrs on 2nd April 1941, the 180 ton gross Leith-registered steel screw ketch (steam trawler) *Cramond Island*, built in 1910 by Mackie & Thomson of Glasgow, engine by W.V.V. Ligerwood of Glasgow, was sunk in error by British aircraft 120° 5 miles off St. Abbs Head.

FORTUNA

Wreck No :	7	Date Sunk :	02 04 1941
Latitude :	55 52 30 N	Longitude :	02 00 00 W
Decca Lat :	5552.50 N	Decca Long :	0200.00 W
Location :	Off St. Abbs Head 120°	Area :	St. Abbs
Type :	Trawler	Tonnage :	259 gross
Length :	128.4 feet Beam : 22.0 feet	Draught :	11.8 feet
How Sunk :	By aircraft	Depth :	64 metres

The 259 ton gross Grimsby steam trawler *Fortuna*, built in 1906 by Cook, Welton & Gemmell of Beverley, was sunk in error by British aircraft 120° off St. Abbs Head on 2nd April 1941. The bodies of two members of her crew were washed ashore at Berwick on 5/4/1941.

ALFRED ERLANDSEN

Wreck No :	8	Date Sunk :	02 10 1907
Latitude :	55 53 42 N	Longitude :	02 07 14 W
Decca Lat :	5553.70 N	Decca Long :	0207.23 W
Location :	Ebb Carrs Rock, St. Abbs	Area :	St. Abbs
Type :	Steamship	Tonnage :	954 gross
Length :	208.0 feet Beam : 31.0 feet	Draught :	14.1 feet
How Sunk :	Ran aground	Depth :	15 metres

In dense fog on the night of Thursday 17th October 1907, the steamship *Alfred Erlandsen*, en route to Grangemouth from Libau in Denmark with a cargo of pit props, ran aground on

Ebb Carrs Rocks off St. Abbs. The ship's whistle alerted the villagers to the plight of the vessel, but in the darkness and thick fog, nothing could be seen of the ship. At that time, St. Abbs had no lifeboat or other rescue apparatus.

The Eyemouth lifeboat, two miles to the South, was called out, as was the Skateraw lifeboat, some twelve miles to the North West. Rocket apparatus was also sent by horse-

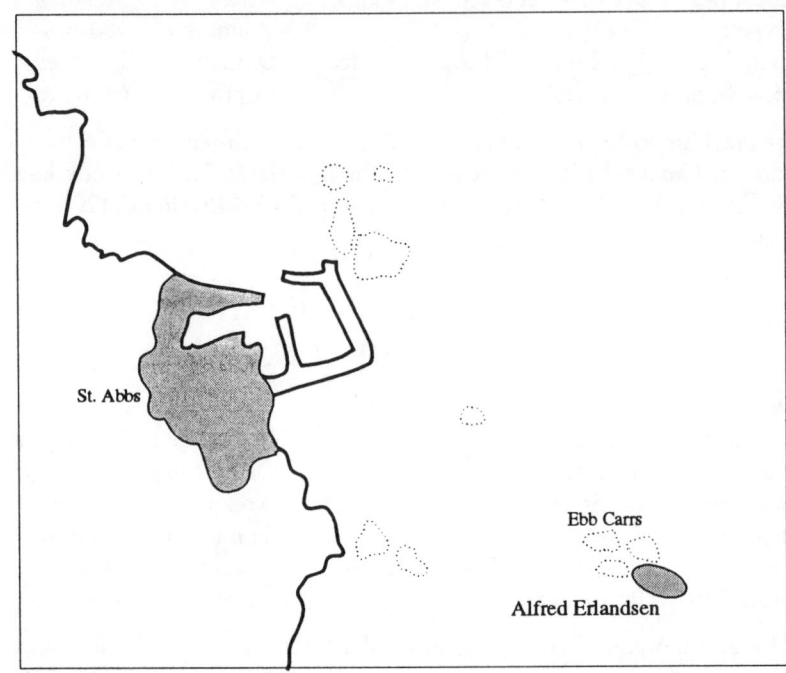

The location of the Alfred Erlandsen near St. Abbs

drawn cart from Eyemouth, but by the time it arrived, the ship's whistle had been silenced by the in-rushing water flooding the furnaces. Although numerous attempts were made to fire a line to the distressed vessel, the rockets did not have sufficient range, and all fell short.

The lifeboats had no engines and had to be rowed through the heavy Easterly swell, the Skateraw boat taking four hours to reach the scene. By that time the *Alfred Erlandsen* and her crew of sixteen had disappeared beneath the surface, and all that remained were the pit props and other floating debris being hurtled around like battering rams by the waves, to the great danger of the lifeboats.

As there were no survivors left to save, the lifeboats headed home. By the time the Skateraw lifeboat returned to her base, she had been at sea for ten hours.

In the morning, however, one survivor, a Great Dane dog was found wandering the cliff tops, having made it ashore through the surf. The dog lived for many years thereafter, and helped to raise money for the Red Cross during the first world war, as the incredible tale of his survival was related over and over again.

As a direct result of the *Alfred Erlandsen* disaster, a lifeboat station was established at St. Abbs in 1911, funded mainly by the Usher Brewery family who lived in the village.

TILLYCORTHIE

Wreck No :	9	**Date Sunk :**	01 03 1917
Latitude :	55 53 50 N PA	**Longitude :**	01 44 00 W PA
Decca Lat :	5553.83 N	**Decca Long :**	0144.00 W
Location :	13 miles E of St. Abbs	**Area :**	St. Abbs
Type :	Steamship	**Tonnage :**	382 gross
Length :	138.6 feet **Beam :** 26.4 feet	**Draught :**	9.9 feet
How Sunk :	Submarine - gunfire	**Depth :**	68 metres

The 382 ton steamship *Tillycorthie* was captured by a submarine and sunk by gunfire on 13th March 1917. Her Master was taken prisoner.

Charted as Wk PA, 13 miles E of St. Abbs Head. *British Vessels Lost At Sea 1939-45* gives the position as 16 miles N $^1/_2$E from Longstone.

BEN SCREEL

Wreck No :	10	**Date Sunk :**	25 12 1942
Latitude :	55 54 00 N PA	**Longitude :**	02 05 00 W PA
Decca Lat :	5554.00 N	**Decca Long :**	0205.00 W
Location :	1.5 miles E of St. Abbs	**Area :**	St. Abbs
Type :	Trawler	**Tonnage :**	195 gross
Length :	115.3 feet **Beam :** 22.1 feet	**Draught :**	11.9 feet
How Sunk :	Mined	**Depth :**	42 metres

The *Ben Screel* (ex-*Gertrude Cappleman*) was a steam trawler built in 1915 by Hall Russell of Aberdeen. The Lat/Long position is doubtful. *British Vessels Lost At Sea 1939-45* merely states "Presumed mined off St. Abbs Head about 25th December 1942".

She had been attacked twice before - the first time on 2nd June 1941, when she was bombed at 5530N, 0130W, and the second time on 12th November 1941 when she was bombed 14 miles North East by North of St. Abbs Head.

ODENSE

Wreck No:	11	Date Sunk:	05 05 1917
Latitude:	55 54 44 N	Longitude:	02 09 12 W
Decca Lat:	5554.73 N	Decca Long:	0209.20 W
Location:	Pettico Wick, St. Abbs Head	Area:	St. Abbs
Type:	Steamship	Tonnage:	1756 gross
Length:	261.0 feet Beam: 36.0 feet	Draught:	16.7 feet
How Sunk:	By U-Boat	Depth:	10 metres

Odense was a 1756 tons gross Danish steamship captured and sunk by a U-Boat on 5th May 1917. She is known as *The Peanut Boat* and lies in Pettico Wick, the bay to the East of St. Abbs Head.

The wreck is completely broken up, with plates and ribs covered in kelp. Her boiler stands vertically in 12 metres.

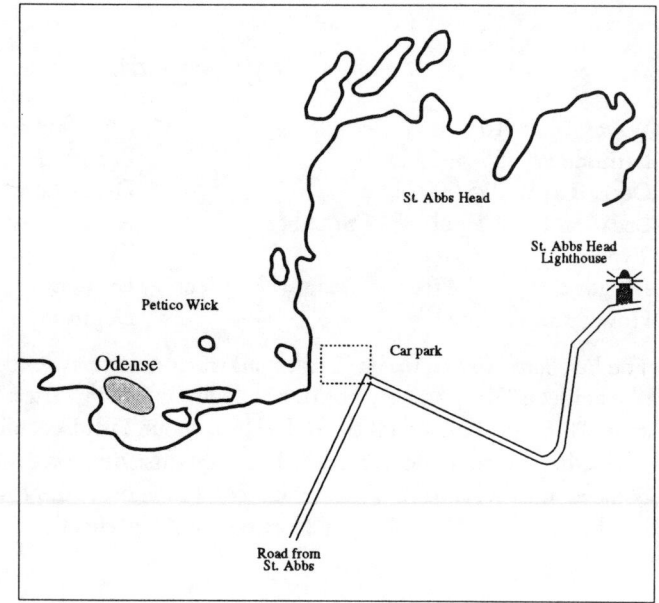

The location of the Odense, or Peanut Boat, in Pettico Wick

BEAR

Wreck No:	12	Date Sunk:	11 01 1891
Latitude:	55 55 00 N PA	Longitude:	02 06 00 W PA
Decca Lat:	5555.00 N	Decca Long:	0206.00 W
Location:	1.25 miles E of St. Abbs Head	Area:	St. Abbs
Type:	Steamship	Tonnage:	596 gross

Length :	174.4 feet	Beam : 25.6 feet	Draught : 14.3 feet
How Sunk :	Collision		Depth : 63 metres

The steamship *Bear* was built in 1877 by R. Dixon & Co. of Middlesbrough, and was sunk in a collision off St. Abbs Head on 11th January 1891. Thirteen of the crew were lost. The position has been estimated from the description "off St. Abbs Head".

AURIAC

Wreck No :	13	Date Sunk :	23 04 1917
Latitude :	55 55 00 N PA	Longitude :	01 50 00 W PA
Decca Lat :	5555.00 N	Decca Long :	0150.00 W
Location :	5 miles ESE from St. Abbs Head	Area :	St. Abbs
Type :	Steamship	Tonnage :	871 gross
Length :	200.0 feet Beam : 29.3 feet	Draught :	15.2 feet
How Sunk :	Submarine - gunfire	Depth :	70 metres

The 871 tons gross steamship *Auriac* (ex-*Adare*, ex-*Taff*), was built by Osbourne, Graham & Co., Sunderland in 1890, and registered in Leith. She was en route from Rouen to Leith in ballast when she was captured and sunk by gunfire by the *UC-44*. One crew member was lost.

Peter Collings gives the position 555700N, 013500W which is 19 miles East of St. Abbs Head. Ian Whittaker gives the wreck charted at 555500N, 015000W PA as *Auriac* and this is 10 miles ESE of St. Abbs Head. Two wrecks are charted 7 miles ESE of St. Abbs Head at 555500N, 015600W, which may be the *Egholm*, and 555530N, 015600W, half a mile further North. *British Vessels Lost at Sea 1914-1918* gives the position of attack as 5 miles ESE from St. Abbs Head, which would result in a PA of 555300N, 020000W. The nearest charted wreck is at 555500N, 015600W (PA), 3 miles from the position of attack.

STRATHRANNOCH

Wreck No :	14	Date Sunk :	06 04 1917
Latitude :	55 55 00 N PA	Longitude :	02 07 00 W PA
Decca Lat :	5555.00 N	Decca Long :	0207.00 W
Location :	0.75 miles E of St. Abbs Head	Area :	St. Abbs
Type :	Trawler	Tonnage :	215 gross
Length :	117.7 feet Beam : 22.1 feet	Draught :	12.2 feet
How Sunk :	Mined	Depth :	44 metres

The *Strathrannoch* was a steel screw ketch (steam trawler), built in 1917 by Hall Russell of Aberdeen. She was requisitioned for use as a mine sweeper during the first world war, and was mined and sunk off St. Abbs Head on 6th April 1917.

GLANMIRE

Wreck No :	15	Date Sunk :	25 07 1912
Latitude :	55 55 02 N	Longitude :	02 08 07 W
Decca Lat :	5555.03 N	Decca Long :	0208.12 W
Location :	300 metres off St. Abbs Head	Area :	St. Abbs
Type :	Steamship	Tonnage :	1141 gross
Length : 242.2 feet	Beam : 33.2 feet	Draught :	15.3 feet
How Sunk :	Ran aground	Depth :	30 metres

The 1141 ton steamship *Glanmire* was built in 1888 by W.B. Thompson of Dundee. While en route from Amsterdam to Grangemouth in thick fog, she struck Black Carrs Rock at about 06.20 am on 25th July 1912, then drifted off to sink half an hour later in 30 metres,

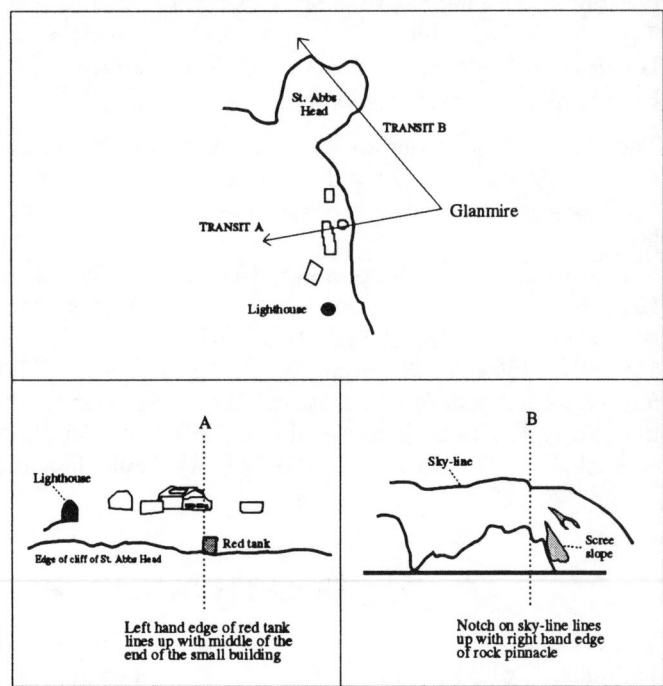

Location of and transits for the Glanmire, off St. Abbs Head

about 300 metres North of St. Abbs Head lighthouse. Her 15 passengers and 22 crew reached shore safely in two boats. The position has been recorded as 555514N, 020812W.

The boilers are still recognisable, but the rest of the wreck is broken up and covered in soft corals, lying on a flat gravel bottom.

TRANSIT A: Line up left hand edge of red tank at lighthouse with centre of gable end of small building attached to large building.
TRANSIT B: To the North East, line up notch on skyline with right hand edge of rock pinnacle.

NYON

Wreck No : 16	Date Sunk : 17 11 1958
Latitude : 55 55 54 N	Longitude : 02 12 48 W
Decca Lat : 5555.90 N	Decca Long : 0212.80 W
Location : Between Souter and Fast Castle	Area : St. Abbs
Type : Motor vessel	Tonnage : 5058 gross
Length : 420.0 feet Beam : 57.0 feet	Draught : 28.0 feet
How Sunk : Ran aground	Depth : 18 metres

Three tugs, the St. Abbs lifeboat and fishing boats from Eyemouth were all involved in salvage efforts after the 5058 tons gross Swiss vessel *Nyon* ran aground North of St. Abbs Head. Despite attempts to plug the holes in her hull with concrete she remained firmly aground by the bow.

The stern half was salved and towed to Holland where a new bow was built on. The rebuilt vessel finally sank some years later in the English Channel. The bow section to aft of the bridge broke up and now lies scattered on the seabed at the foot of the cliffs.

It may still be possible to see the remains of lifting tackle installed at the top of the cliff during the salvage attempts.

GASRAY

Wreck No : 17	Date Sunk : 05 04 1945
Latitude : 55 56 00 N PA	Longitude : 02 09 00 W PA
Decca Lat : 5556.00 N	Decca Long : 0209.00 W
Location : 2 miles N3/4E St. Abbs Head	Area : St. Abbs
Type : Steamship	Tonnage : 1406 gross
Length : 234.3 feet Beam : 36.3 feet	Draught : feet
How Sunk : Torpedoed	Depth : 60 metres

The 1406 tons gross British steamship *Gasray* was torpedoed on 5th April 1945, 2 miles N 3/4 E from St. Abbs Head, while en route from Grangemouth to Blyth. Of the 18 crew and 4 gunners, 6 crew members were lost.

MAGICIENNE

Wreck No :	18	Date Sunk :	04 05 1940
Latitude :	55 56 06 N	Longitude :	02 19 45 W
Decca Lat :	5556.10 N	Decca Long :	0219.75 W
Location :	N. end of Pease Bay	Area :	St. Abbs
Type :	Schooner	Tonnage :	250 gross
Length :	116.3 feet Beam : 27.2 feet	Draught :	12.8 feet
How Sunk :	Ran aground	Depth :	2 metres

The 250 ton 3-masted wooden schooner *Magicienne* was built at St. Malo in 1912. She had an auxiliary 2-cylinder oil engine.

She ran aground on 4th May 1940, and part of the wreck is visible at low tide close to the rocks at the North end of the sandy beach at Pease Bay.

DOVE

Wreck No :	19	Date Sunk :	Pre-1919
Latitude :	55 56 30 N PA	Longitude :	02 16 00 W PA
Decca Lat :	5556.50 N	Decca Long :	0216.00 W
Location :	1.5 miles NW of Fast Castle	Area :	St. Abbs
Type :	Trawler	Tonnage :	168 gross
Length :	118.0 feet Beam : 20.7 feet	Draught :	10.9 feet
How Sunk :		Depth :	28 metres

Two vessels named Dove appear in Lloyds Register of Shipping:
- *Dove* (Trawler)-iron screw ketch, 168 tons gross, 118 x 20.7 x 10.9 feet, built 1877 by Edwards Bros. North Shields, engine by N.E. Marine of Sunderland. Registered in Hull. (Reg. No. H1033). This *Dove* sank in the North Sea during a hurricane on 6th March 1883.
- *Dove* (Whaler)-steel screw steamer 128 tons gross, 100.4 x 18.4 x 10.8 feet, built in 1911 by Framnaes Mek. Vaerks, Sandefjord, engine by Fredrikstad MV. It is not known why, where, or even if this *Dove* sank.

The wreck charted PA, 1.5 miles NW of Fast Castle was reported in 1919, and either of the *Dove* s above would seem possible, but when the wreck is found, recovered parts such as the engine makers plate should establish her true identity.

See the wreck at 560310N, 021650W which is an apparently accurate position for a wreck fairly close to the obviously approximate position given for the *Dove* .

Berwick, Eyemouth, St. Abbs & Dunbar

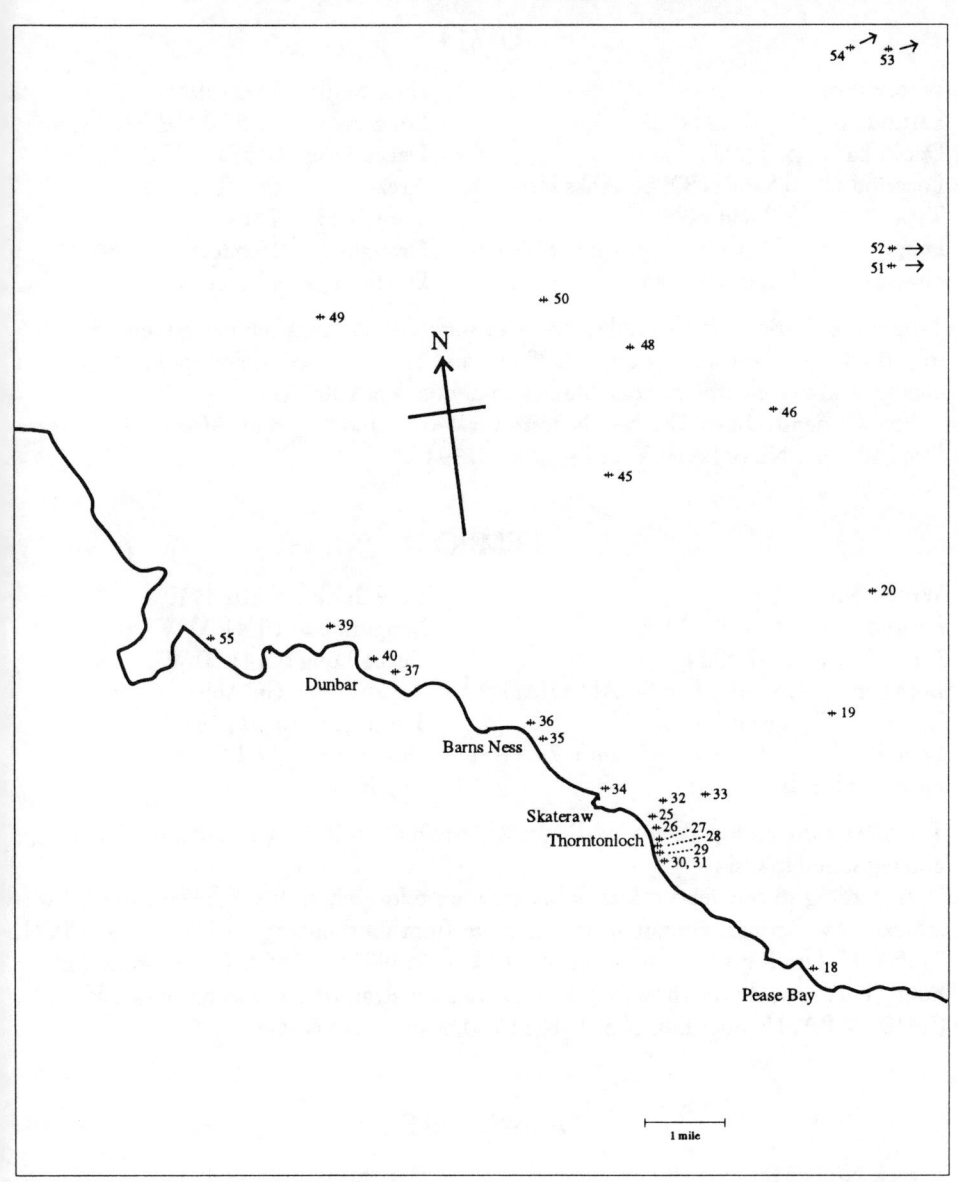

Chart of the location of wrecks to the South of and around Dunbar

U-714

Wreck No :	20	Date Sunk :	14 03 1945
Latitude :	55 57 00 N PA	Longitude :	01 57 00 W PA
Decca Lat :	5557.00 N	Decca Long :	0157.00 W
Location :	6.5 miles 80° St. Abbs Head	Area :	St. Abbs
Type :	Submarine	Tonnage :	761 gross
Length :	221.0 feet Beam : 20.5 feet	Draught :	15.8 feet
How Sunk :	Depth charged	Depth :	73 metres

Type V11C U-Boat, 761 tons displacement surfaced, 865 tons submerged. Fitted with 5 torpedo tubes, 4 bow and 1 stern, 1 x 88 mm and 1 x 20 mm guns. Powered by two diesel engines and two electric motors. Maximum diving depth 309 feet

She was depth charged by the RN destroyer *Wyvern* and the South African Navy frigate *Natal* 10 miles NE of Berwick on 14th March 1945.

TEMPO ?

Wreck No :	21	Date Sunk :	03 02 1940
Latitude :	55 57 30 N PA	Longitude :	01 41 00 W PA
Decca Lat :	5557.50 N	Decca Long :	0141.00 W
Location :	15 miles E of St. Abbs Head	Area :	St. Abbs
Type :	Steamship	Tonnage :	629 gross
Length :	178.7 feet Beam : 29.5 feet	Draught :	12.2 feet
How Sunk :	By aircraft	Depth :	60 metres

The 629 ton steamship *Tempo* (ex-*Borgsvold*), was built in 1903 by P. Larsson of Thorskog, and registered in Oslo.

According to one report, five of her crew were lost when this Norwegian vessel was attacked by German aircraft while en route from Gothenburg to Hull, at 560900N, 013500W. *Lloyds* give the position of attack as 555900N, 013500W, ten miles further South, but it is not known how long she remained afloat, and the wreck charted at 555730N, 014100W PA, 15 miles East of St. Abbs Head, may be the *Tempo*.

DUNSCORE ?

Wreck No :	22	Date Sunk :	05 12 1934
Latitude :	55 58 12 N	Longitude :	02 01 06 W
Decca Lat :	5558.20 N	Decca Long :	0201.10 W
Location :	5 miles ENE of St. Abbs Head	Area :	St. Abbs
Type :	Steamship	Tonnage :	176 gross
Length :	100.0 feet Beam : 20.1 feet	Draught :	8.3 feet
How Sunk :		Depth :	74 metres

A wreck is charted in this position 5 miles ENE of St. Abbs Head, and may be the *Dunscore*, a 176 tons gross iron-hulled steel screw steamship built in 1898 by J. McArthur & Co., Paisley, engine by Bow, McLachlan of Paisley.

VERBORMILIA

Wreck No :	23	**Date Sunk :**	06 02 1940
Latitude :	56 00 00 N PA	**Longitude :**	02 14 00 W PA
Decca Lat :	5600.00 N	**Decca Long :**	0214.00 W
Location :	4 miles N of Fast Castle Head	**Area :**	St. Abbs
Type :	Steamship	**Tonnage :**	3275 gross
Length :	331.0 feet **Beam :** 48.3 feet	**Draught :**	22.0 feet
How Sunk :	Ran aground	**Depth :**	58 metres

It has been suggested that an unknown WW2 loss dating from before March 1945 lies in this approximate position. The nearest known wartime loss to this position was the steamship *Verbormilia*, and this may have been an administratively convenient *parking place* to represent the loss of that vessel on 6th February 1940.

If there is a wreck in this position, 4 miles from the shore, North of Fast Castle Head, it is unlikely to be the *Verbormilia*, as she was reported to be stranded West of Fast Castle. I would suggest around 555600N, 021400W, close to the shore near Nick Cove would be a better place to start searching for her.

Verbormilia (ex-*Danubio*), built in 1907 by W. Gray & Co., Hartlepool, was the only ship owned by the Verbormilia Steamship Co. of London. A vessel of this size so close to the shore must be worth searching for.

Pease Bay, 3 miles to the West, or St. Abbs, 5 miles to the South East, are the nearest launching sites for this otherwise inaccessible stretch of cliff-lined coast.

UTOPIA

Wreck No :	24	**Date Sunk :**	10 08 1915
Latitude :	56 00 00 N PA	**Longitude :**	01 49 30 W PA
Decca Lat :	5600.00 N	**Decca Long :**	0149.50 W
Location :	12 miles E of St. Abbs Head	**Area :**	St. Abbs
Type :	Steamship	**Tonnage :**	155 gross
Length :	100.0 feet **Beam :** 19.8 feet	**Draught :**	10.0 feet
How Sunk :	Submarine gunfire	**Depth :**	49 metres

Utopia was captured by a U-Boat 12 miles E of St. Abbs Head on 10th August 1915, and sunk by gunfire. Charted as Wreck PA.

ABERAVON

Wreck No :	25	Date Sunk :	05 02 1878
Latitude :	55 57 45 N PA	Longitude :	02 23 00 W PA
Decca Lat :	5557.75 N	Decca Long :	0223.00 W
Location :	Thorntonloch, 2.5 miles E of Dunbar	Area :	Dunbar
Type :	Steamship	Tonnage :	382 gross
Length :	feet Beam : feet	Draught :	feet
How Sunk :	Ran aground	Depth :	metres

The 382 ton iron steamship *Aberavon*, en route from Middlesbrough to Grangemouth with a cargo of pig iron, ran aground at Thorntonloch, 2.5 miles East of Dunbar on 5th February 1878, and became a total loss.

JOHN

Wreck No :	26	Date Sunk :	11 03 1895
Latitude :	55 57 45 N PA	Longitude :	02 23 00 W PA
Decca Lat :	5557.75 N	Decca Long :	0223.00 W
Location :	Thorntonloch	Area :	Dunbar
Type :	Brig	Tonnage :	280 gross
Length :	feet Beam : feet	Draught :	feet
How Sunk :	Ran aground	Depth :	metres

The 280 ton Norwegian brig *John*, with a cargo of ice (!) from Christiania to Sunderland, was lost on the rocks near Thorntonloch on 11th March 1895.

This was obviously before the days of refrigeration, and I suppose one had to obtain ice somehow when the need was identified. I can confidently state without fear of contradiction that this is one wreck which will be impossible to identify by her cargo!

ANDROMEDA

Wreck No :	27	Date Sunk :	05 01 1911
Latitude :	55 57 45 N PA	Longitude :	02 23 00 W PA
Decca Lat :	5557.75 N	Decca Long :	0223.00 W
Location :	Stranded at Longcraig	Area :	Dunbar
Type :	Schooner	Tonnage :	223 gross
Length :	109.3 feet Beam : 27.2 feet	Draught :	12.0 feet
How Sunk :	Ran aground	Depth :	metres

The Russian 3-masted wooden schooner *Andromeda* stranded at Longcraig on 5th January 1911 while en route from London to Bo'ness with a cargo of scrap iron. She was built at Riga in 1900.

KING JAJA

Wreck No : 28	Date Sunk : 13 10 1905
Latitude : 55 57 45 N PA	Longitude : 02 23 00 W PA
Decca Lat : 5557.75 N	Decca Long : 0223.00 W
Location : Stranded at Longcraig	Area : Dunbar
Type : Steamship	Tonnage : 201 gross
Length : 125.3 feet Beam : 19.8 feet	Draught : 9.3 feet
How Sunk : Ran aground	Depth : 5 metres

On 14th October 1905, the Methil steamship *King Jaja*, bound from Newcastle to Methil with a cargo of steel rails, got into difficulties near Dunbar in a violent Northerly gale, and was driven ashore. Dunbar lifeboat went to her assistance, but the *King Jaja* got off under her own steam. Later, however, she was driven ashore again, and the lifeboat put out a second time. This time, the *King Jaja*'s position was critical, and she could not be refloated.

King Jaja was built in 1870 by J. & R. Swan of Glasgow.

AGNES

Wreck No : 29	Date Sunk : 29 07 1898
Latitude : 55 57 45 N PA	Longitude : 02 23 00 W PA
Decca Lat : 5557.75 N	Decca Long : 0223.00 W
Location : Longcraig Rocks, Thorntonloch	Area : Dunbar
Type : Brig	Tonnage : 266 gross
Length : feet Beam : feet	Draught : feet
How Sunk : Ran aground	Depth : metres

The 266 ton Norwegian brig *Agnes*, from Drammen to Bo'ness with a cargo of pit props, was blown on to Longcraig reef at Thorntonloch by a NNE gale on 29th July 1898.

CYDUM

Wreck No : 30	Date Sunk : 01 11 1905
Latitude : 55 57 45 N PA	Longitude : 02 23 00 W PA
Decca Lat : 5557.75 N	Decca Long : 0223.00 W
Location : Lunciwick, Thorntonloch	Area : Dunbar
Type : Schooner	Tonnage : 100 gross
Length : feet Beam : feet	Draught : feet
How Sunk : Ran aground	Depth : metres

Shortly after 9.00 pm on 1st November 1905, the schooner *Cydum* was blown ashore during a wild North Easterly gale and torrents of rain on the Lunciwick, between Thorntonloch and Cockburnspath. Immediate assistance was needed as the vessel was in great peril. In the darkness and very heavy sea, the Dunbar lifeboat was launched. Dunbar rocket brigade also drove to the scene and succeeded in rescuing the crew of the *Cydum* before the lifeboat arrived. It appeared the *Cydum* was blown into the bay and struck the rocks which run out to sea for a long distance. The vessel rapidly broke up in the heavy seas. The *Cydum* had been en route from Southampton to Dysart in ballast.

PROSUM

Wreck No :	31	Date Sunk :	24 10 1908
Latitude :	55 57 45 N PA	Longitude :	02 23 00 W PA
Decca Lat :	5557.75 N	Decca Long :	0223.00 W
Location :	Longcraig Rocks, Thorntonloch	Area :	Dunbar
Type :	Steamship	Tonnage :	684 gross
Length :	200.0 feet Beam : feet	Draught :	feet
How Sunk :	Ran aground	Depth :	5 metres

The 684 tons net Norwegian iron steamship *Prosum* ran ashore at Longcraig, Thorntonloch, near Dunbar on 24th October, 1908 while en route from London to Grangemouth. She broke in two after running on to the Bathe Reef.

It has been reported that only a winch assembly remains, but perhaps the diver who reported this merely failed to find other wreckage, of which there must be a substantial amount in the area, as quite a number of vessels have been lost here over the years.

LIVLIG

Wreck No :	32	Date Sunk :	06 03 1919
Latitude :	55 58 00 N PA	Longitude :	02 22 00 W PA
Decca Lat :	5558.00 N	Decca Long :	0222.00 W
Location :	Between Cove and Torness	Area :	Dunbar
Type :		Tonnage :	277 gross
Length :	118.8 feet Beam : 26.4 feet	Draught :	13.2 feet
How Sunk :	Foundered	Depth :	11 metres

The *Livlig* foundered abreast St. Abbs Head, $1/2$ mile offshore on 6th March 1919.

RIVER GARRY

Wreck No :	33	Date Sunk :	18 11 1893
Latitude :	55 58 00 N PA	Longitude :	02 22 00 W PA
Decca Lat :	5558.00 N	Decca Long :	0222.00 W
Location :	1 mile E of Torness Power Stn	Area :	Dunbar
Type :	Steamship	Tonnage :	1294 gross
Length :	240.0 feet Beam : 33.2 feet	Draught :	18.2 feet
How Sunk :	Foundered in a hurricane	Depth :	30 metres

The 1294 ton steamship *River Garry* was built in 1883 by Workman Clark of Belfast. Her crew of 19 were all lost when she foundered in a Force 12 NNE hurricane off Goatness Point near Dunbar on 18th November 1893, while en route from Leith to London with a cargo of coal. Her broken up remains lie on a rock and shingle bottom at 26-30 metres.

RIBNITZ

Wreck No :	34	Date Sunk :	21 09 1891
Latitude :	55 58 42 N PA	Longitude :	02 25 00 W PA
Decca Lat :	5558.70 N	Decca Long :	0225.00 W
Location :	Skateraw	Area :	Dunbar
Type :	Schooner	Tonnage :	270 gross
Length :	feet Beam : feet	Draught :	feet
How Sunk :	Ran aground	Depth :	metres

The German schooner *Ribnitz*, en route from Riga to Bo'ness with a cargo of pit props, was dashed on to the rocks at Skateraw by a North Easterly storm on 21st September 1891.

SCANDIA

Wreck No :	35	Date Sunk :	21 09 1891
Latitude :	55 59 00 N PA	Longitude :	02 26 00 W PA
Decca Lat :	5559.00 N	Decca Long :	0226.00 W
Location :	Eastbarns, S of Barns Ness	Area :	Dunbar
Type :	Barque	Tonnage :	335 gross
Length :	feet Beam : feet	Draught :	feet
How Sunk :	Ran aground	Depth :	metres

On 21st September 1891, the 335 ton Norwegian barque *Scandia*, en route from Sundswall to Grangemouth with a cargo of battens, was blown on to the rocks at Eastbarns in a North Easterly storm.

ECCLEFECHAN

Wreck No :	36	Date Sunk :	23 02 1900
Latitude :	55 59 42 N	Longitude :	02 26 24 W
Decca Lat :	5559.70 N	Decca Long :	0226.40 W
Location :	0.5 miles NE of Barns Ness	Area :	Dunbar
Type :	Barque	Tonnage :	2105 gross
Length :	290.7 feet Beam : 42.2 feet	Draught :	23.8 feet
How Sunk :	Ran aground	Depth :	8 metres

In 1959, HMS *Egeria* reported a wreck about 2 cables SE of the Ruddystone, half a mile North East of Barns Ness. There is a considerable compass anomaly in this area, probably caused by the presence of a great amount of iron. Boat-shaped lead ingots have been recovered from the wreck, which is charted as Wk PA.

The 2031 ton net Glasgow-registered iron-hulled barque *Ecclefechan*, built by R. Duncan of Port Glasgow in 1882, was en route from Chittagong to Dundee with a cargo of jute when she was lost near Skateraw Rocks on 23rd February 1900.

STELLA MARIS

Wreck No :	37	Date Sunk :	13 08 1877
Latitude :	56 00 00 N PA	Longitude :	02 29 30
Decca Lat :	5600.00 N	Decca Long :	0229.50 W
Location :	½ mile E of Vault Point	Area :	Dunbar
Type :	Schooner	Tonnage :	118 gross
Length :	feet Beam : feet	Draught :	feet
How Sunk :	Ran aground	Depth :	metres

In a Force 5 North Easterly wind on 13th August 1877, the 118 ton Dutch schooner *Stella Maris*, bound from Gothenburg to South Alloa with a cargo of battens, was lost by stranding on the rocks half a mile East of Vault Point, Dunbar.

UNKNOWN

Wreck No :	38	Date Sunk :	
Latitude :	56 00 30 N PA	Longitude :	02 13 00 W PA
Decca Lat :	5600.50 N	Decca Long :	0213.00 W
Location :	6 miles N of St. Abbs Head	Area :	Dunbar
Type :		Tonnage :	
Length :	feet Beam : feet	Draught :	feet
How Sunk :		Depth :	60 metres

Charted as Wk PA in 60 metres.

FOX

Wreck No :	39	Date Sunk :	14 11 1745
Latitude :	56 00 30 N PA	Longitude :	02 30 30 W PA
Decca Lat :	5600.50 N	Decca Long :	0230.50 W
Location :	Off Dunbar	Area :	Dunbar
Type :	6th rate Man o' War	Tonnage :	
Length : feet	Beam : feet	Draught :	feet
How Sunk :		Depth :	12 metres

HMS Fox is reputed to have been loaded with valuables belonging to local landowners fleeing from advancing English forces after the battle of Prestonpans in 1745. Cannon have been found in the area, along with timbers of appropriate age.

FRIGGA

Wreck No :	40	Date Sunk :	20 12 1876
Latitude :	56 00 30 N PA	Longitude :	02 30 24 W PA
Decca Lat :	5600.50 N	Decca Long :	0230.40 W
Location :	1/2 mile E of Dunbar Harbour	Area :	Dunbar
Type :	Barque	Tonnage :	334 gross.
Length : feet	Beam : feet	Draught :	feet
How Sunk :		Depth :	metres

The 334 ton Norwegian barque *Frigga*, en route, in ballast, from Berwick to Brevig, was dashed on to the rocks $1/_2$ mile East of Dunbar Harbour in an ESE storm on 20th December 1876.

UNKNOWN

Wreck No :	41	Date Sunk :	WW2
Latitude :	56 01 30 N PA	Longitude :	02 05 30 W PA
Decca Lat :	5601.50 N	Decca Long :	0205.50 W
Location :	6.5 miles NNE St. Abbs Head	Area :	Dunbar
Type :		Tonnage :	
Length : feet	Beam : feet	Draught :	feet
How Sunk :	Ran aground	Depth :	10 metres

There is thought to be an unknown WW2 loss in this approximate position.

UNKNOWN

Wreck No :	42	Date Sunk :	WW2
Latitude :	56 02 00 N PA	Longitude :	02 12 00 W PA
Decca Lat :	5602.00 N	Decca Long :	0212.00 W
Location :	PA 6 miles NNE of Fast Castle	Area :	Dunbar
Type :		Tonnage :	
Length : feet	Beam : feet	Draught :	feet
How Sunk :		Depth :	62 metres

The wreck charted in 62 metres at 560200N, 021200W PA, 6 miles NNE of Fast Castle is thought to be an unknown WW2 loss.

HALLAND

Wreck No :	43	Date Sunk :	15 09 1940
Latitude :	56 03 00 N PA	Longitude :	02 17 00 W PA
Decca Lat :	5603.00 N	Decca Long :	0217.00 W
Location :	70° 8 miles from Dunbar	Area :	Dunbar
Type :	Steamship	Tonnage :	1264 gross
Length : 238.0 feet	Beam : 37.2 feet	Draught :	13.7 feet
How Sunk : Bombed		Depth :	53 metres

The steamship *Halland* was built in 1923 at Keil, and registered in Copenhagen. She was attacked by aircraft while en route from London to Dundee with 1900 tons of cement. Seventeen of the crew of 22 were lost. The trawler *Sparta* took surviving crew members to Methil.

UNKNOWN - ADORATION ?

Wreck No :	44	Date Sunk :	Pre 03 1919
Latitude :	56 03 10 N	Longitude :	02 16 50 W
Decca Lat :	5603.17 N	Decca Long :	0216.83 W
Location :	70° 8 miles from Dunbar	Area :	Dunbar
Type :		Tonnage :	
Length : feet	Beam : feet	Draught :	feet
How Sunk :		Depth :	50 metres

An unknown wreck sunk pre-1919 is charted in this position. It may be the *Adoration*, which sank in March 1919, or possibly the *Dove*.

CYCLOPS

Wreck No:	45	**Date Sunk:**	21 02 1924
Latitude:	56 03 43 N	**Longitude:**	02 29 38 W
Decca Lat:	5603.72 N	**Decca Long:**	0229.63 W
Location:	2.8 miles 96° from Bass Rock	**Area:**	Dunbar
Type:	Dredger	**Tonnage:**	
Length: 180.0 feet	**Beam:** 25.0 feet	**Draught:**	7.0 feet
How Sunk:	Foundered	**Depth:**	34 metres

The dredger *Cyclops* sank en route from Queensferry to Sunderland to be scrapped, and is now lying broken up in approximately 41 metres, standing up 5 or 6 metres from the bottom, and lying NNE/SSW. The wreck is charted at 560343N, 022938W, 3.5 miles NNE of Dunbar.

UNKNOWN - WW2 ?

Wreck No:	46	**Date Sunk:**	WW2
Latitude:	56 04 00 N PA	**Longitude:**	02 21 00 W PA
Decca Lat:	5604.00 N	**Decca Long:**	0221.00 W
Location:	5.5 miles NW of Barns Ness	**Area:**	Dunbar
Type:		**Tonnage:**	
Length: feet	**Beam:** feet	**Draught:**	feet
How Sunk:		**Depth:**	50 metres

An unknown WW2 wreck is thought to lie in this approximate position. Could this be the *Cradock*? Another possibility is that this may be the 50 ton iron dredger *Scotia* which foundered about 7 miles off Dunbar on 21st September 1893 while en route from Eyemouth to Granton in a Force 6 North Easterly.

CRADOCK

Wreck No:	47	**Date Sunk:**	08 11 1941
Latitude:	56 05 00 N PA	**Longitude:**	02 00 00 W PA
Decca Lat:	5605.00 N	**Decca Long:**	0200.00 W
Location:	11 miles NNE of St. Abbs Head	**Area:**	Dunbar
Type:	Trawler	**Tonnage:**	204 gross
Length: 115.4 feet	**Beam:** 22.2 feet	**Draught:**	12.1 feet
How Sunk:	Bombed	**Depth:**	55 metres

The *Cradock* was a steam trawler built in 1919 by Hawthorns & Co. of Leith and registered in North Shields.
    She was bombed and machine-gunned by a JU-88 at 18.30 hrs on 8th November 1941. *British Vessels Lost at Sea 1939-1945* gives the position of attack as 14 miles NNE of St. Abbs

Head. According to *Lloyds* she was abandoned 12 miles NE of St. Abbs Head and is presumed to have sunk. The nine crewmen were all saved.

A wreck is charted at 560500N, 020000W PA, which is 11 miles NNE of St. Abbs Head, and may be an official estimate of the sinking position of the *Cradock*.

UNKNOWN

Wreck No :	48	Date Sunk :	
Latitude :	56 05 20 N	Longitude :	02 24 53 W
Decca Lat :	5605.33 N	Decca Long :	0224.88 W
Location :	6 miles NE of Dunbar	Area :	Dunbar
Type :		Tonnage :	
Length :	feet Beam : feet	Draught :	feet
How Sunk :		Depth :	45 metres

This position is 7 miles 150° from the May Island, which, taking into account the annual magnetic variation in the area, coincides with the description of the position given in *British Vessels Lost At Sea 1914-18* for the loss of the *Sabbia* in 1916, but the wreck in this position is only 100 feet long, whereas the *Sabbia* was 315 feet long. (See *Sabbia* at 560612N, 022518W, $^3/_4$ mile from this position).

MORESBY

Wreck No :	49	Date Sunk :	Pre-1919
Latitude :	56 06 01 N	Longitude :	02 31 07 W
Decca Lat :	5606.02 N	Decca Long :	0231.12 W
Location :	4 miles E of Bass Rock	Area :	Dunbar
Type :	Steamship	Tonnage :	1763 gross
Length :	260.8 feet Beam : 34.6 feet	Draught :	24.0 feet
How Sunk :		Depth :	40 metres

Built in 1881 by R. Dixon & Co. of Middlesbrough, the *Moresby* (ex-*Jacob Christensen*), appears in *Lloyds Register* 1912-13.

She was reported in this position on 24th March 1919, by the Senior Naval Officer at Granton, but according to *Dictionary of Disasters at Sea in the Age of Steam*, the *Moresby* was torpedoed and sunk by the *U-39* 120 miles NW by W of Alexandria, Egypt at 32 36N, 28 38E on 28th November 1916, with the loss of 33 of her crew. She had been en route from Saigon to Dunkirk with a cargo of rice

SABBIA

Wreck No :	50	Date Sunk :	20 04 1916
Latitude :	56 06 12 N	Longitude :	02 25 18 W
Decca Lat :	5606.20 N	Decca Long :	0225.30 W
Location :	6.5 miles NW of Dunbar	Area :	Dunbar
Type :	Steamship	Tonnage :	2807 gross
Length :	314.6 feet Beam : 46.8 feet	Draught :	13.7 feet
How Sunk :	Mined	Depth :	44 metres

In 1968, in 560600N, 022500W PA, an unidentified wreck was thought to originate from WW2. A more accurate position has since been established, and the wreck is now charted at 560612N, 022518W, 6.25 miles 150° from the May Island.

This is very close to the position given for the loss of the *Sabbia* in 1916, which was described as 7 miles SE by S from the May Island, (i.e. 145° from the May Island), in *British Vessels Lost At Sea 1914-18*. The annual magnetic variation in the area decreases by 4 minutes, resulting in a 1990 bearing of 150° from the May Island, along which the Lat/Long position given above lies.

The *Sabbia* was a steel screw steamer built in 1903 by R. Stephenson & Co. of Newcastle, and registered in London. She hit one of 34 mines laid by *U-74* (Weisbach).

BOYNE CASTLE

Wreck No :	51	Date Sunk :	07 02 1917
Latitude :	56 07 00 N PA	Longitude :	02 09 00 W PA
Decca Lat :	5607.00 N	Decca Long :	0209.00 W
Location :	12 miles N by E of St. Abbs Head	Area :	Dunbar
Type :	Steamship	Tonnage :	245 gross
Length :	118.8 feet Beam : 23.1 feet	Draught :	6.6 feet
How Sunk :	Submarine-gunfire	Depth :	58 metres

The position description given in *British Vessels Lost At Sea 1914-18* is 12 miles N by E of St. Abbs Head, which suggests a PA of 560700N, 020900W. Ian Whittaker gives 560636N, 020400W, 2.75 miles away, (uncharted).

The nearest charted wreck (PA) is less than $^1/_2$ a mile away at 560718N, 020920W but this is reputedly the *Pathfinder*.

There are several unknown wrecks charted within a few miles of the derived position for the *Boyne Castle*. How accurate was the original position description? Did the *Boyne Castle* sink immediately, or did she perhaps drift for a time before sinking?

PATHFINDER

Wreck No :	52	Date Sunk :	05 09 1914
Latitude :	56 07 18 N	Longitude :	02 09 20 W
Decca Lat :	5607.30 N	Decca Long :	0209.33 W
Location :	14 miles ESE of May Island	Area :	Dunbar
Type :	Light cruiser	Tonnage :	2940 gross
Length :	379.0 feet Beam : 38.5 feet	Draught :	13.0 feet
How Sunk :	Torpedoed by *U-21*	Depth :	58 metres

The wreck charted as PA at 560718N, 020920W is known to local fishermen as the destroyer *Pathfinder*, built in 1904 by Cammell Laird of Birkenhead. The 1919 report gave the approximate position as 560800N, 020500W. HMS *Pathfinder* was the first warship to be sunk by a torpedo fired from a submarine.

The destroyer's forward magazine blew up when she was torpedoed by the *U-21*, (Hersing), and she sank in four minutes with the loss of 259 of the 268 crew.

The first merchantman sunk by a submarine, (but not by torpedoing), was the British steamship *Glitra*, (ex-*Saxon Prince*), 866 tons gross, 215 x 31 x 14 feet, built in 1895 by R & W Hawthorn of Newcastle, and belonging to Christian Salvesen of Leith. On 20th October 1914, while en route from Grangemouth to Stavanger, and while awaiting a pilot 14 miles WSW of Skudesnes, she was captured by the *U-17* (Feldkirchner), who appeared on the surface.

The crew were given 10 minutes to leave the ship before she was scuttled by the Germans after the *Glitra*'s crew were safely in their lifeboats.

ZZ 12

Wreck No :	53	Date Sunk :	05 05 1946
Latitude :	56 09 00 N	Longitude :	02 13 07 W
Decca Lat :	5609.00 N	Decca Long :	0213.12 W
Location :	14 miles NNE of St. Abbs Head	Area :	Dunbar
Type :	Mine sweeper	Tonnage :	360 gross
Length :	145.0 feet Beam : 30.0 feet	Draught :	2.2 feet
How Sunk :	Foundered	Depth :	58 metres

This is the ZZ 12, a Z-Class Lighter (Landing Craft), converted in late 1944 to a mine sweeper, which capsized and sank while under tow on 5th May 1946. She was powered by two diesel engines.

KITTY

Wreck No :	54	**Date Sunk :**	09 05 1917
Latitude :	56 11 39 N PA	**Longitude :**	01 45 00 W PA
Decca Lat :	5611.65 N	**Decca Long :**	0145.00 W
Location :	25 miles ENE St. Abbs Head	**Area :**	Dunbar
Type :	Trawler	**Tonnage :**	181 gross
Length :	105.0 feet **Beam :** 21.0 feet	**Draught :**	11.2 feet
How Sunk :	Submarine-bomb	**Depth :**	52 metres

The steel screw ketch (steam trawler) *Kitty* was built by Earle's Co., Hull in 1898 and registered in Fleetwood.

There is also another *Kitty* in the 1916-17 *Lloyds Register of Shipping* - a steel screw steamship of 135 tons gross, 96.7 x 20.1 x 10.5 feet built by A. Hall & Co., Aberdeen in 1897, and registered in Aberdeen. She was captured by a U-Boat and sunk by explosive charge 25 miles ENE of St. Abbs Head. Her skipper and chief engineer were taken as prisoners.

The nearest charted wreck is shown at 561139N, 024500W PA, 21 miles ENE of St. Abbs Head.

CHAPTER 3

THE WRECKS OF NORTH BERWICK, ABERLADY & LEITH

INTRODUCTION

This area, which covers the south shore of the Forth estuary, is rocky at its eastern end, around North Berwick, giving way towards the west to a gently-sloping, low-lying coast with large sandy areas. Unfortunately, the only place at which a boat may be launched is North Berwick.

The distance by water from North Berwick to the western parts of the area is so great, however, that it would be more practical to launch from the north shore of the Forth to reach some of the wrecks in this area.

The Bass Rock lies almost two miles offshore and is 320 feet high. It holds the world's largest gannetry. The lighthouse, which is about 150 feet. above sea level, was built in 1902, and its beam is visible for 18 miles. A tunnel running North west - South east through the rock is accessible at low tide.

The barren, rocky islands of Craigleith, and Lamb also lie off North Berwick. They are inhabited by numerous seabirds. Although no vessels have been lost on them, they provide interesting scenic diving.

Fidra, whose name means *Feather Island*, is owned by the Royal Society for the Protection of Birds, and is a breeding place for eider duck. It also has a lighthouse toward its North end.

Robert Louis Stevenson is said to have been inspired by horseshoe-shaped Fidra when he wrote *Treasure Island*, while living in North Berwick.

The old trading village of Aberlady was a small port until its channel to the sea silted up in the 1850s and created a wide sandy bay. This now forms a nature reserve noted for its birds and butterflies. Aberlady now provides convenient accommodation for those sampling the nature reserve and local golf course.

Leith is the major port in the Forth which covers some 600 acres. It provides extensive modern commercial docking facilities for much of the South east of Scotland. Granton and Newhaven are much smaller ports also near to Edinburgh Unlike Leith, they provide facilities, such as launching slips for small vessels.

North Berwick, Aberlady & Leith

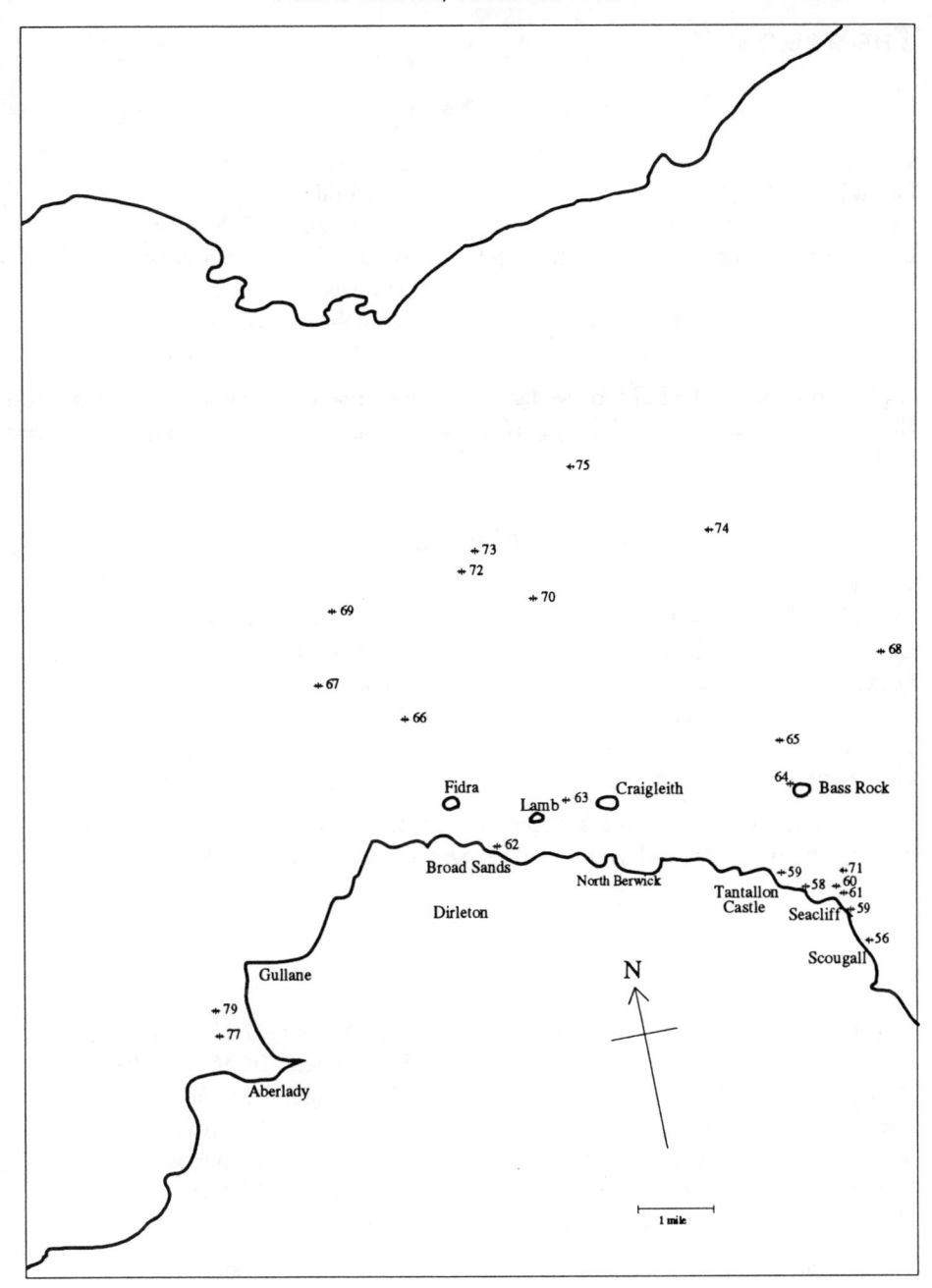

Chart showing the location of wrecks lying North of the coast stretching between Aberlady and Scoughall on the South coast of the Firth of Forth

The Wrecks

HIRAM

Wreck No :	55	Date Sunk :	29 02 1916
Latitude :	56 01 42 N	Longitude :	02 35 15 W
Decca Lat :	5601.70 N	Decca Long :	0235.25 W
Location :	Frances Craig, Scougall Rocks	Area :	North Berwick
Type :	Brig	Tonnage :	507 gross
Length :	138.6 feet Beam : 33.0 feet	Draught :	16.5 feet
How Sunk :	Ran aground	Depth :	18 metres

All 12 of the crew of the 507 ton Swedish barque *Hiram* were lost when she ran aground on Hedderwick Sands on 29th February 1916 while carrying a cargo of pit props from Drammen to Blyth.

SOPHIE

Wreck No :	56	Date Sunk :	21 09 1891
Latitude :	56 02 30 N PA	Longitude :	02 36 30 W PA
Decca Lat :	5602.50 N	Decca Long :	0236.50 W
Location :	Scougall Rocks	Area :	North Berwick
Type :	Schooner	Tonnage :	139 gross
Length :	feet Beam : feet	Draught :	feet
How Sunk :	Ran aground	Depth :	metres

In a North Easterly storm on 21st September 1891, the 139 ton Danish schooner *Sophie*, bound from Svendborg to Dysart in ballast, was lost on Scougall Rocks.

PODEROSA

Wreck No :	57	Date Sunk :	27 11 1896
Latitude :	56 03 00 N PA	Longitude :	02 36 30 W PA
Decca Lat :	5603.00 N	Decca Long :	0236.50 W
Location :	Seacliff, Scougall Rocks	Area :	North Berwick
Type :	Steamship	Tonnage :	1183 gross
Length :	249.8 feet Beam : 32.9 feet	Draught :	19.9 feet
How Sunk :	Ran aground	Depth :	7 metres

The iron steamship *Poderosa*, built in 1875 by Cole Bros., ran aground while en route, in ballast, from Grimsby to Grangemouth. She was 732 tons net.

ELTERWATER

Wreck No :	58	Date Sunk :	08 08 1927
Latitude :	56 03 06 N	Longitude :	02 36 48 W
Decca Lat :	5603.10 N	Decca Long :	0236.80 W
Location :	The Rodgers, Scougall Rocks	Area :	North Berwick
Type :	Steamship	Tonnage :	2126 gross
Length :	280.5 feet Beam : 42.9 feet	Draught :	9.9 feet
How Sunk :	Ran aground	Depth :	7 metres

The Newcastle steamship *Elterwater* ran aground in dense fog near South Carr Rock on Saturday 6th Aug 1927 while bound from Antwerp to Grangemouth with a cargo of pig iron. Two women and two men went ashore in the vessel's own boat. Dunbar lifeboat stood by the steamer, but the remaining crew would not leave, hoping that they might be refloated. Badly holed and taking in much water, the steamer's fore part was almost awash at high water. Salvage was to commence immediately. Memories of shipwreck obviously fade fairly quickly, and are not well-recorded, as only 32 years later, in 1959, this was reported as an unknown stranded and heavily salvaged wreck at Seacliff, South of North Berwick

VALHALLA

Wreck No :	59	Date Sunk :	27 02 1900
Latitude :	56 03 20 N PA	Longitude :	02 38 45 W PA
Decca Lat :	5603.33 N	Decca Long :	0238.75 W
Location :	Near Tantallon Castle	Area :	North Berwick
Type :	Barque	Tonnage :	477 gross
Length :	feet Beam : feet	Draught :	feet
How Sunk :	Ran aground	Depth :	metres

The Norwegian iron barque *Valhalla*, en route from London to Dundee in ballast was driven ashore near Tantallon Castle by a Force 10 North Easterly storm on 27th February 1900.

THOMAS ALFRED

Wreck No :	60	Date Sunk :	23 10 1881
Latitude :	56 03 24 N PA	Longitude :	02 37 30 W PA
Decca Lat :	5603.40 N	Decca Long :	0237.50 W
Location :	South Carr Rock	Area :	North Berwick
Type :	Brig	Tonnage :	204 gross
Length :	feet Beam : feet	Draught :	feet
How Sunk :	Ran aground	Depth :	metres

The 204 ton Norwegian brig *Thomas Alfred* was blown on to South Carr Rock in a severe ESE storm on 23rd October 1881.

MARIA

Wreck No : 61
Latitude : 56 03 24 N PA
Decca Lat : 5603.40 N
Location : Near South Carr Rocks
Type : Schooner
Length : feet **Beam :** feet
How Sunk : Ran aground

Date Sunk : 31 08 1876
Longitude : 02 37 30 W PA
Decca Long : 0237.50 W
Area : North Berwick
Tonnage : 173 gross
Draught : feet
Depth : metres

The 173 ton Faversham schooner Maria was blown on to the rocks near South Carr Rock in a Force 10 North Easterly storm while en route from Ramsgate to Burntisland in ballast on 31st August 1876. She was a total loss.

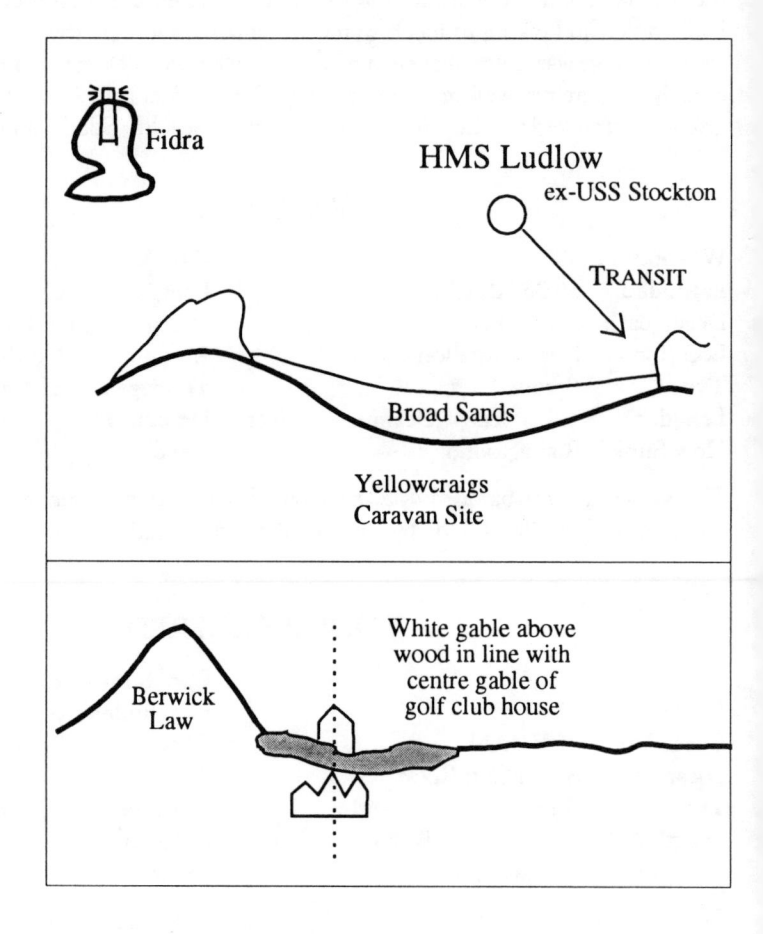

Sketch of the location and transit for HMS Ludlow, which was used as a target in Broad Sands

LUDLOW

Wreck No :	62	Date Sunk :	05 07 1945
Latitude :	56 03 55 N	Longitude :	02 45 58 W
Decca Lat :	5603.92 N	Decca Long :	0245.97 W
Location :	Broad Sands, Dirleton	Area :	North Berwick
Type :	Destroyer	Tonnage :	1020 gross
Length :	315.5 feet Beam : 30.5 feet	Draught :	7.5 feet
How Sunk :	Aircraft rocket target	Depth :	7 metres

HMS *Ludlow* (ex-*USS Stockton*), built in 1917 by Wm. Cramp, was one of 50 WW1 destroyers given to Britain in 1940 by the USA in exchange for the U.S. having the right to establish military bases in various British possessions, mainly in the Caribbean and Bermuda, under an agreement of 2/9/1940. After being scrapped on 5/7/1945, the vessel was used as a rocket target by the RAF.

She has been extensively salvaged, and lies partly buried in sand a few hundred yards off the beach at Dirleton. Her bows break the surface at low water.

BULL

Wreck No :	63	Date Sunk :	06 12 1893
Latitude :	56 04 30 N PA	Longitude :	02 43 00 W PA
Decca Lat :	5604.50 N	Decca Long :	0243.00 W
Location :	Between Lamb and Craigleith	Area :	North Berwick
Type :	Steamship	Tonnage :	522 gross
Length :	feet Beam : feet	Draught :	feet
How Sunk :	Collision with *Rosslyn*	Depth :	15 metres

The steamship *Bull* was sunk after being struck amidships in a collision with the Leith steam trawler *Rosslyn* about 1 mile from North Berwick, between Craigleith and Lamb. She was en route from Grangemouth to Middlesbrough with four passengers, but otherwise in ballast. One member of the crew of the *Rosslyn* was lost. A weather report in the *Fifeshire Advertiser* of 6/12/1893 noted that a violent storm of West wind had been blowing over this district during the greater part of the week, accompanied by drizzling rain.

General depths in the area range from 14-19 metres to a sandy bottom. I have searched between the two islands, and the area between the islands and North Berwick fairly thoroughly by echo-sounder, but found nothing. The wreck must lie slightly further North of a straight line between the islands, as presumably she had set a course to pass outside the islands.

UNKNOWN

Wreck No :	64	Date Sunk :	1905
Latitude :	56 04 45 N PA	Longitude :	02 38 30 W PA
Decca Lat :	5604.75 N	Decca Long :	0238.50 W
Location :	Close W of Bass Rock	Area :	North Berwick
Type :		Tonnage :	
Length : feet	Beam : feet	Draught :	feet
How Sunk :		Depth :	30 metres

This wreck was first reported in the *Underwater World* magazine of May 1967, lying in 30 metres, off the North West corner of the Bass Rock, suggesting that she may have struck the Bass.

Statistical details of ships lost around Scotland in 1905 were published in *Parliamentary Papers* dated 1907. Appended to these papers is a map showing the positions of the 1905 losses. One of the wreck positions is marked immediately adjacent to the Bass Rock, but unfortunately, the map is of such a small scale that it is not possible to determine the exact position, and the vessel is not identified in the accompanying text.

STELLA

Wreck No :	65	Date Sunk :	08 12 1903
Latitude :	56 05 00 N PA	Longitude :	02 38 00 W PA
Decca Lat :	5605.00 N	Decca Long :	0238.00 W
Location :	Near the Bass Rock	Area :	North Berwick
Type :	Steamship	Tonnage :	198 gross
Length : feet	Beam : feet	Draught :	feet
How Sunk :	Collision with *Waterland*	Depth :	metres

The 198 ton Norwegian steel steamship *Stella*, bound from Burntisland to Haugesund, was sunk in a collision with the Dutch steamship *Waterland* near the Bass Rock on 8th December 1903. Three of her crew were lost.

UNKNOWN - 1930s ?

Wreck No :	66	Date Sunk :	Pre-1979
Latitude :	56 05 14 N	Longitude :	02 49 43 W
Decca Lat :	5605.23 N	Decca Long :	0249.72 W
Location :	1.5 miles NW of Fidra	Area :	North Berwick
Type :	Steamship	Tonnage :	
Length : feet	Beam : feet	Draught :	feet
How Sunk :		Depth :	28 metres

First located 14/12/1979, this is reputedly a collier lost off Fidra in the 1930s. It is reported in the *Kingfisher Book of Tows Vol. 1* in Decca Chain 3, as Green C 38.90, Purple C 61.00.

UNKNOWN - PRE 1979

Wreck No :	67	Date Sunk :	Pre-1979
Latitude :	56 06 06 N	Longitude :	02 50 06 W
Decca Lat :	5606.10 N	Decca Long :	0250.10 W
Location :	3 miles NW of Fidra	Area :	North Berwick
Type :		Tonnage :	
Length : feet	Beam : feet	Draught :	feet
How Sunk :		Depth :	51 metres

First located 14/12/1979 in Decca Chain 3, Green C38.50, Purple C63.10 (*Kingfisher Book of Tows Vol. 1*).

ROYAL FUSILIER

Wreck No :	68	Date Sunk :	03 06 1941
Latitude :	56 06 32 N	Longitude :	02 35 18 W
Decca Lat :	5606.53 N	Decca Long :	0235.30 W
Location :	2.4 miles NE of Bass Rock	Area :	North Berwick
Type :	Steamship	Tonnage :	2187 gross
Length : 290.2 feet	Beam : 41.2 feet	Draught :	18.0 feet
How Sunk : Bombed		Depth :	40 metres

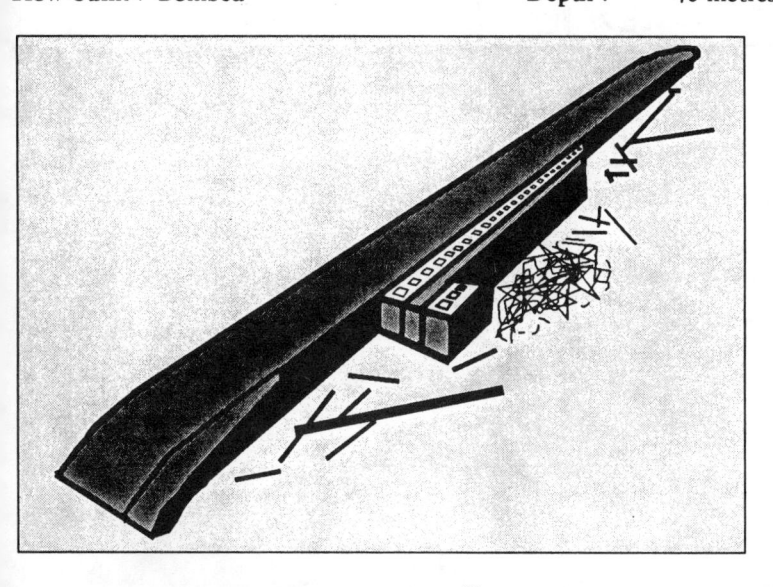

Sketch of the Royal Fusilier lying on her port side in some 40 metres of water

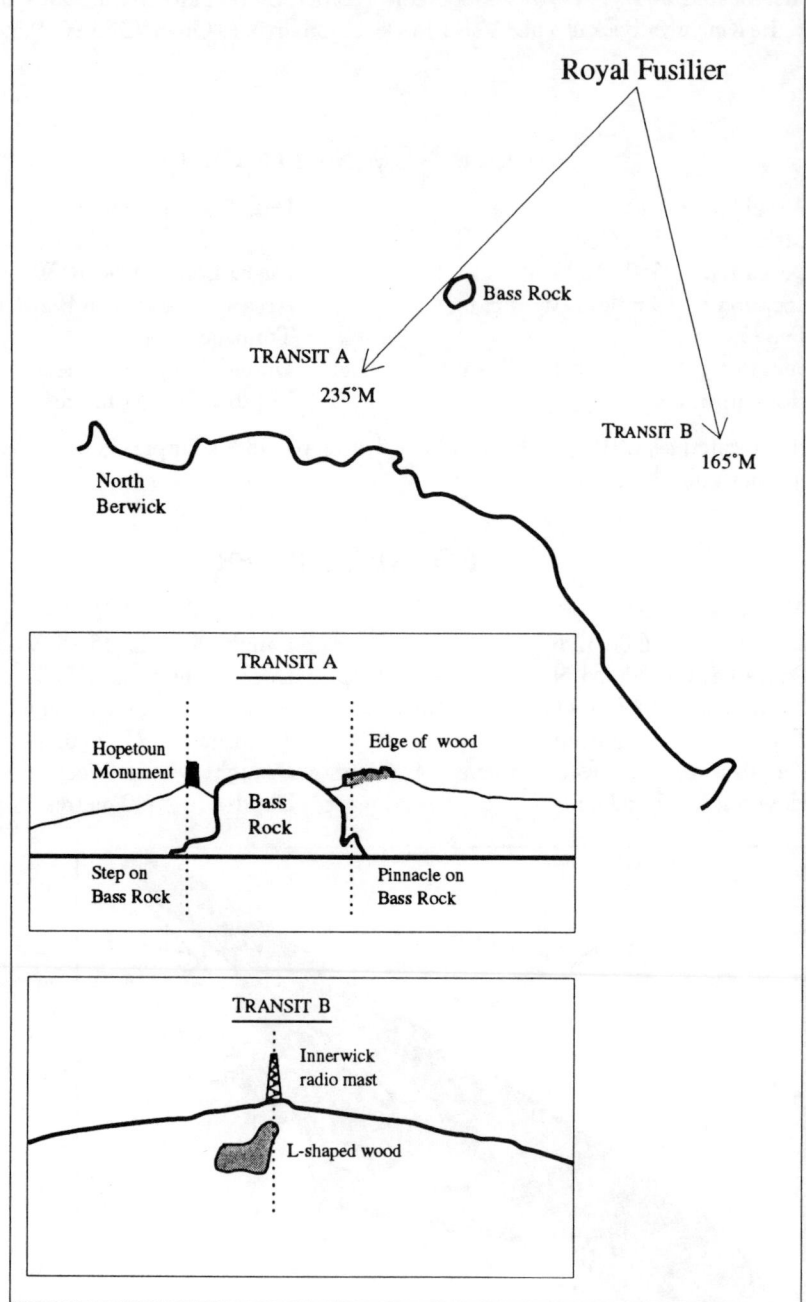

Sketch of the location of and transits for the Royal Fusilier, near Bass Rock

The *Royal Fusilier* was built in 1924 by Caledon of Dundee, and registered in Leith. She was bombed at 5522N, 0121W while en route from London to Leith with a cargo of 50 tons of rice and 70 tons of paper. The damaged vessel was taken in tow, but capsized and sank at 4.18 pm at 560648N, 023500W. Her crew of 27 were all saved.

The wreck is now lying on its port side, half buried in the mud.

DUNA ?

Wreck No :	69		Date Sunk :	03 02 1902
Latitude :	56 06 59 N		Longitude :	02 49 18 W
Decca Lat :	5606.98 N		Decca Long :	0249.30 W
Location :	2.7 miles NNW of Fidra		Area :	North Berwick
Type :	Schooner		Tonnage :	119 gross
Length :	feet	Beam : feet	Draught :	feet
How Sunk :	Collision with *Chancellor*		Depth :	51 metres

This wreck was first located by HMS *Scott* in 1959, and charted in the above position in 55 metres of water. It stands up 4 metres from the bottom, and therefore its least depth is 51 metres. This position is 4 miles SSW of Elie, but it is also 2.7 miles NNW of Fidra. The magnetic variation in the area would have been much greater in 1902, and at that time the bearing would have been almost NW of Fidra.

On 3rd February 1902, the Norwegian schooner *Duna* was sunk in collision with the Granton steamer *Chancellor* about 3 miles NW of Fidra. The *Duna* was en route, in ballast, from Egersund to West Wemyss, and two lives were lost.

UNKNOWN

Wreck No :	70		Date Sunk :	
Latitude :	56 07 00 N		Longitude :	02 45 42 W
Decca Lat :	5607.00 N		Decca Long :	0245.70 W
Location :	2.7 miles NNE of Fidra		Area :	North Berwick
Type :			Tonnage :	
Length :	feet	Beam : feet	Draught :	feet
How Sunk :			Depth :	56 metres

An unknown wreck is charted at 560700N, 024542W with at least 28 metres over it in about 56 metres. This is 2.7 miles NNE of Fidra.

ELIZA

Wreck No :	71	Date Sunk :	02 10 1899
Latitude :	56 03 24 N PA	Longitude :	02 37 30 W PA
Decca Lat :	5603.24 N	Decca Long :	0237.50 W
Location :	South Carr Beacon, Seacliff	Area :	North Berwick
Type :	Barque	Tonnage :	447 gross
Length :	feet Beam : feet	Draught :	feet
How Sunk :	Ran aground	Depth :	7 metres

The Danish iron barque *Eliza* struck the rocks at the South Carr beacon, off Seacliff on 2nd October 1899, with the loss of 10 lives. She had been en route from Bremerhaven to Methil in ballast.

MUNCHEN

Wreck No :	72	Date Sunk :	1921
Latitude :	56 07 18 N	Longitude :	02 46 21 W
Decca Lat :	5607.30 N	Decca Long :	0246.35 W
Location :	2.9 miles N of Fidra	Area :	North Berwick
Type :	Light cruiser	Tonnage :	3756 gross
Length :	364.7 feet Beam : 43.7 feet	Draught :	18.4 feet
How Sunk :	Torpedo experiment	Depth :	50 metres

Built by Weser in 1905, and disarmed in 1916, the German light cruiser *Munchen* was assigned to Britain in 1920 for scrap, but it is not known whether any scrapping work was actually done before she was expended in a torpedo experiment in 1921. As the disarming of the ship was carried out by the Germans themselves in 1916, this presumably included the removal of the guns, for which they no doubt had rather pressing alternative use in the middle of the First World War.

Charted as Wk in the above position with a clearance of at least 28 metres in about 56 metres depth.

UNKNOWN - PRE 1935

Wreck No :	73	Date Sunk :	Pre-1935
Latitude :	56 07 31 N	Longitude :	02 49 04 W
Decca Lat :	5607.52 N	Decca Long :	0249.07 W
Location :	3.5 miles S of Elie	Area :	North Berwick
Type :		Tonnage :	
Length :	feet Beam : feet	Draught :	feet
How Sunk :		Depth :	36 metres

The wreck charted 3.5 miles South of Elie at 560731N, 024904W (36 metres in 49 metres), was first located in 1935, and reported in 1959 by HMS Scott to have a least depth of 120 feet, standing some 34 feet above the sea bed, indicating that it must be a fairly substantial vessel

This may be the *Stjernvik*. This position is also 339° 3.41 miles from Fidra lighthouse, and the wreck is known to some of the local fishermen as *"Tommy Littles"*.

Compare this with the reports of the *Avondale Park* (2878 tons, standing up 32 feet from the bottom), and the *Rolfsborg* (1825 tons, standing up 40 feet).

STJERNVIK

Wreck No :	74	Date Sunk :	12 04 1928
Latitude :	56 07 45 N	Longitude :	02 41 00 W
Decca Lat :	5607.75 N	Decca Long :	0241.00 W
Location :	3 miles N of Bass Rock	Area :	North Berwick
Type :	Steamship	Tonnage :	1174 gross
Length :	240.0 feet Beam : 34.2 feet	Draught :	14.1 feet
How Sunk :	Collision	Depth :	40 metres

Stjernvik was an iron screw steamship built in 1883 by Barrow S.B. Co., and registered in Sweden.

She was in collision in dense fog with the British steamship *British Ambassador* on 12th April 1928 off Fidra while en route from Ridham Dock to Burntisland in ballast.

The Swedish vessel was badly damaged, and the crew took to their boats, where they remained until the *Stjernvik* disappeared. They were then taken aboard the *British Ambassador* and landed in Leith. The *British Ambassador* was en route in ballast from Grangemouth to the Tyne, and was able to continue on its voyage.

UNKNOWN - PRE 1962

Wreck No :	75	Date Sunk :	Pre-1962
Latitude :	56 08 17 N	Longitude :	02 44 46 W
Decca Lat :	5608.28 N	Decca Long :	0244.77 W
Location :	3.5 miles SE of Elie	Area :	North Berwick
Type :		Tonnage :	
Length :	feet Beam : feet	Draught :	feet
How Sunk :		Depth :	48 metres

First located in 1962 by the survey ship *HMS Scott*, standing up 4 metres in 52 metres.

UNKNOWN - BARGE

Wreck No :	76	Date Sunk :	WW2
Latitude :	56 00 42 N	Longitude :	02 56 20 W
Decca Lat :	5600.70 N	Decca Long :	0256.33 W
Location :	Gosford Bay, 3 miles Cockenzie	Area :	Aberlady
Type :	Barge	Tonnage :	
Length :	feet Beam : feet	Draught :	feet
How Sunk :		Depth :	6 metres

The wreck charted at 560042N, 025620W in Gosford Bay, 3 miles off Cockenzie, is reported to be a barge which sank during WW2.

UNKNOWN X-CRAFT

Wreck No :	77	Date Sunk :	04 1946
Latitude :	56 01 21 N	Longitude :	02 52 45 W
Decca Lat :	5601.35 N	Decca Long :	0252.75 W
Location :	Aberlady Bay	Area :	Aberlady
Type :	Submarine X-Craft	Tonnage :	30 gross
Length :	51.6 feet Beam : 5.8 feet	Draught :	7.4 feet
How Sunk :	Scuttled	Depth :	0 metres

Another X-Craft midget submarine lies fairly close by at 560126N, 025309W.

The width dimension is for the X-Craft without its two side charges, each of which contained about 2 tons of explosive, detonated by clockwork time fuses. It was possible for a diver to leave and return to the submerged craft to place the charges on the bottom, under the ship to be attacked.

The two X-Craft midget submarines in Aberlady Bay were placed there in April 1946, to be used as bombing or rocket targets for practice by low-flying aircraft, in the same way as the destroyer HMS *Ludlow* (ex-*USS Stockton*), a few miles further East. In the late 1940s they were known locally as "*The 20s*", and are thought to be two of the following three X-Craft: *X-20*, *X-21* or *X-25*.

Some years ago, the non-ferrous metal was salvaged by someone who drove a tractor over the sands to the submarines, which are uncovered at low tide, but the bulk of both submarines still lies there, partially buried in the sand.

Around 1960, the author Nigel Tranter, who lives nearby, used the Westernmost of the two submarines as a hide while wildfowling in Aberlady Bay, and became trapped inside when the hatch seized shut. To effect an escape, he used the barrels of his shotgun as a lever to prise the hatch open before the incoming tide completely engulfed the submarine again! This incident was incorporated in a fictionalised account described in his novel *Drug on the Market*, published in 1962. In that book, he describes these submarines as Japanese, but they are in fact British, of the same type used to attack the German battleship *Tirpitz* in Kaafiord,

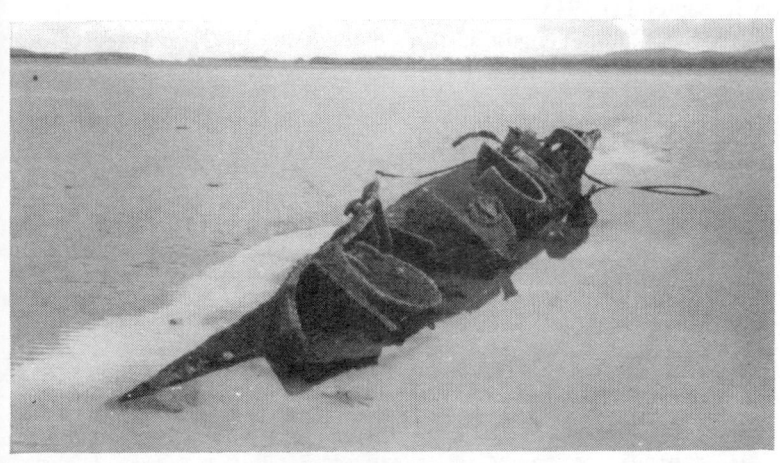

The two X-Craft in Aberlady Bay (Photos by Bob Baird)

The more westerly of the X-Craft seen from the bows

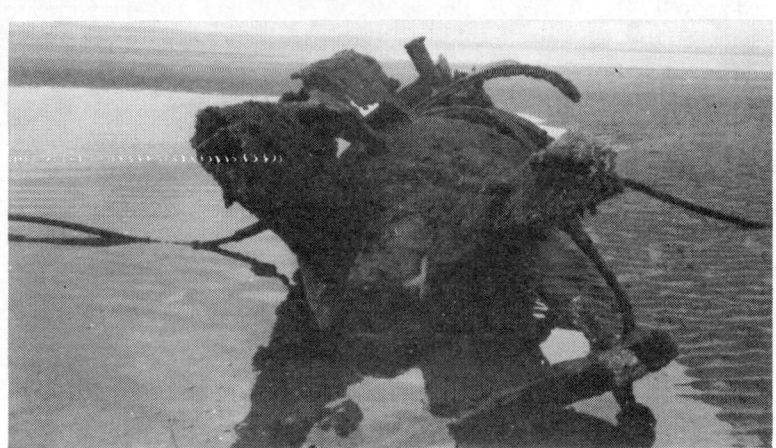

The more westerly of the X-Craft seen from the stern

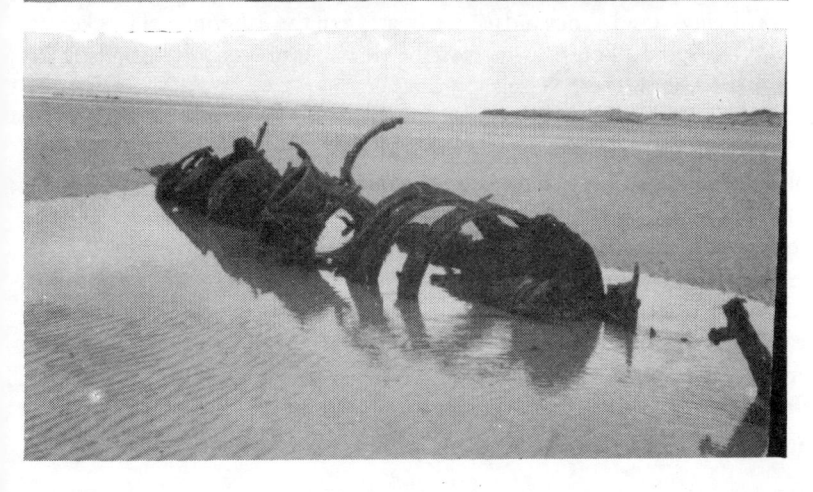

The more easterly and more broken of the X-Craft seen from the port quarter

Northern Norway in September 1943.

They were powered by a Gardner engine and an electric motor, and had a crew of four, although on close examination they seem to have barely enough room inside for one crew member.

UNKNOWN

Wreck No :	78	Date Sunk :	1920-1939?
Latitude :	56 01 24 N	Longitude :	02 57 24 W
Decca Lat :	5601.40 N	Decca Long :	0257.40 W
Location :	3 miles WNW of Aberlady Bay	Area :	Aberlady
Type :	Drifter ?	Tonnage :	
Length :	feet Beam : feet	Draught :	feet
How Sunk :		Depth :	13 metres

The wreck charted at 560124N, 025724W, 3 miles WNW of Aberlady Bay is reported to be a drifter sunk between the two wars. Possibly the *Leonard*?

Wreckage found on the seabed in 1970 measured about 40 feet x 20 feet by 15 feet high.

UNKNOWN

Wreck No :	79	Date Sunk :	
Latitude :	56 01 52 N	Longitude :	02 52 20 W
Decca Lat :	5601.87 N	Decca Long :	0252.33 W
Location :	Aberlady Bay	Area :	Aberlady
Type :	Drifter	Tonnage :	
Length :	feet Beam : feet	Draught :	feet
How Sunk :		Depth :	metres

One of the Earls of Wemyss used to buy old fishing boats from the fishermen of Cockenzie, and dumped them off Kilspindie Point "to improve the view". Paintings of the Aberlady Bay area, dated around 1940, show these vessels.

At 560152N, 025220W, in Aberlady Bay, the remains of the keel and ribs of a wooden vessel partially buried in the sand, uncover at low water. This might be one of these old fishing boats, although it does seem to have been a somewhat larger vessel. The remains of other old wooden boats are shown on the chart at: 560138N, 025233W, and 560044N, 025205W. Aberlady Bay has gradually filled up with sand over the years.

In 1547, Henry VIII sent up a fleet to try to relieve the English Force besieged in Haddington, but these vessels were repelled by the cannon of French mercenaries based at Luffness Castle, at the head of the bay, and had to go over to Fife instead, to wreak vengeance there. Whether any of these ships were sunk is not recorded, but Henry's anger was such that he ordered Luffness to be "spoiled" after the English won the battle of Pinkie (Musselburgh) two years later.

— North Berwick, Aberlady & Leith —

UNKNOWN - PRE 1959

Wreck No : 80
Latitude : 56 02 15 N
Decca Lat : 5602.25 N
Location : 1.5 miles W of Gullane Point
Type : Steamship ?
Length : feet Beam : feet
How Sunk :

Date Sunk : Pre-1959
Longitude : 02 54 33 W
Decca Long : 0254.55 W
Area : Aberlady
Tonnage :
Draught : feet
Depth : 11 metres

The wreck of a *puffer* type vessel was reported here by fishermen in 1959.

LCA 672? OR LCA 811?

Wreck No : 81
Latitude : 56 02 58 N
Decca Lat : 5602.97 N
Location : South Channel
Type : Landing Craft
Length : 41.5 feet Beam : 10.0 feet
How Sunk : Foundered

Date Sunk : 02 04 1944
Longitude : 03 00 15 W
Decca Long : 0300.25 W
Area : Aberlady
Tonnage : 13 gross
Draught : 2.2 feet
Depth : 14 metres

Charted as a wreck at 13.5 metres in a general depth of 17 metres, and classified by the Navy as a Landing Craft which sank in 1944. In 1975, divers estimated her to be standing about 8 feet above the seabed.

Landing Craft LCA 845 of 13.5 tons displacement was also sunk at 560527N, 025312W on 29/1/1944, during exercises off Leith, East Scotland. LCA 552 was wrecked 9/2/1944 during exercises off East Scotland. LCA 672 and LCA 811 foundered during exercises off East Scotland on 2/4/1944.

It is interesting that the word *wrecked* was used in respect of LCA 552, (this can usually be interpreted as *ran aground*), while the word *foundered* was used to describe the circumstances of loss for LCAs 672 and 811. This wreck is therefore likely to be either LCA 672 or LCA 811.

These two landing craft were converted with strengthened hull frames, and were equipped to explode minefields in the path of an assault landing, for which purpose they were armed with 24 mortars in four rows of six.

CHESTER II

Wreck No : 82
Latitude : 56 04 16 N
Decca Lat : 5604.27 N
Location : Gullane Bay
Type : Trawler
Length : 104.0 feet   **Beam :** 21.0 feet
How Sunk : Collision

Date Sunk : 29 02 1916
Longitude : 02 52 15 W
Decca Long : 0252.25 W
Area : Aberlady
Tonnage : 143 gross
Draught : 11.0 feet
Depth : 17 metres

Chester II was an iron-hulled steam trawler built in 1896, and owned by the Consolidated Steam Fishing & Ice Co. Ltd.

The wreck is intact and the holds are full of silt. There are strong tidal streams in this area.

TRANSITS:
1) Left end of Fidra in line with the highest part of the Bass Rock.
2) Left wall of Fidra light in line with right shoulder of the Bass Rock.
3) Hopetoun monument in line with V-shaped tree to right of Gullane House.

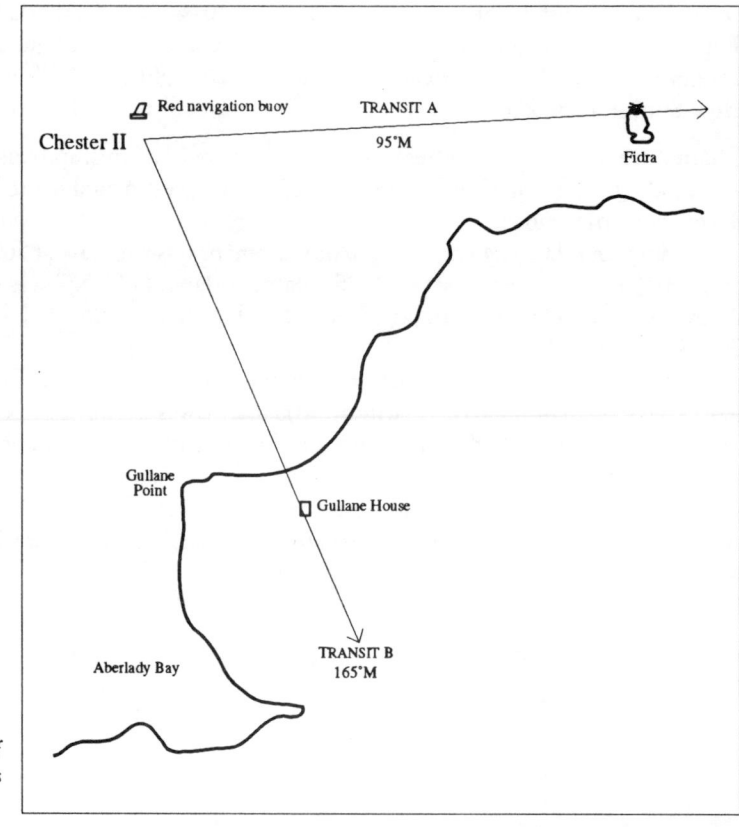

Sketch of the location of the Chester II which lies off Gullane Bay

BARGE G4

Wreck No :	83	Date Sunk :	1953
Latitude :	56 05 15 N	Longitude :	02 55 10 W
Decca Lat :	5605.25 N	Decca Long :	0255.17 W
Location :	3.5 miles NNW of Gullane Point	Area :	Aberlady
Type :	Barge	Tonnage :	
Length :	feet Beam : feet	Draught :	feet
How Sunk :		Depth :	33 metres

The barge G4 was first located by HMS Scott in 1959 in position 560515N, 025513W, standing up 12 feet from the bottom, with a least depth to the wreck of 110 feet The position was given as 560501N, 025503W in 1968, but is now charted at 560515N, 025510W.

The barge was reported to be salvaged in 1953, but it was located by HMS Scott in 1959!

LCA 845

Wreck No :	84	Date Sunk :	29 01 1944
Latitude :	56 05 27 N	Longitude :	02 53 12 W
Decca Lat :	5605.45 N	Decca Long :	0253.20 W
Location :	5 miles N of Gullane Point	Area :	Aberlady
Type :	Landing Craft	Tonnage :	14 gross
Length :	41.5 feet Beam : feet	Draught :	feet
How Sunk :	Foundered	Depth :	38 metres

See the wreck at 560258N, 030015W. LCA 845 became waterlogged and sank during exercises off Leith.

UNKNOWN

Wreck No :	85	Date Sunk :	WW2
Latitude :	55 58 12 N	Longitude :	03 01 32 W
Decca Lat :	5558.20 N	Decca Long :	0301.53 W
Location :	1 mile NW of Musselburgh	Area :	Leith
Type :		Tonnage :	
Length :	feet Beam : feet	Draught :	feet
How Sunk :		Depth :	7 metres

This is thought to be an unknown WW2 wreck.

Another wreck may exist 3 cables to the East of this position.

IVANHOE

Wreck No :	86	Date Sunk :	03 11 1914
Latitude :	55 59 30 N PA	Longitude :	03 10 00 W PA
Decca Lat :	5559.50 N	Decca Long :	0310.00 W
Location :	4 cables, 38° Martello Tower	Area :	Leith
Type :	Trawler	Tonnage :	190 gross
Length :	112.2 feet Beam : 19.8 feet	Draught :	9.9 feet
How Sunk :	Ran aground	Depth :	1 metres

British Vessels Lost At Sea 1914-18 merely states "wrecked in Firth of Forth". *Ivanhoe*, (Trawler No. 664), was stranded 4 cables, 38° from the Martello Tower half a mile East of Leith Docks.

BAYONET

Wreck No :	87	Date Sunk :	21 12 1939
Latitude :	55 59 50 N	Longitude :	03 09 54 W
Decca Lat :	5559.83 N	Decca Long :	0309.90 W
Location :	0.75 miles NW of Leith Docks	Area :	Leith
Type :	Boom Defence	Tonnage :	605 gross
Length :	159.7 feet Beam : 30.7 feet	Draught :	13.0 feet
How Sunk :	Mined	Depth :	8 metres

HMS *Bayonet* (ex-*Barnehurst*), was a Navy lifting vessel of the *Net* class, with bow horns, mined and sunk at 15.00 hrs on 21st December 1939, and reported to lie at 555950N, 030954W, 3/4 mile North West of Leith docks.

No wreck is charted in that position, but an obstruction charted at 560010N, 030940W, 1/4 mile away may be the *Bayonet*.

The sound of the explosion of the mine was heard in Edinburgh, but its cause was not immediately apparent, and was at first thought to be a bomb. RAF fighters were despatched from Drem to search for German bombers, and two RAF Hampden bombers were shot down in error, one of them crashing into the sea off Gullane. The Hampdens were part of a flight from RAF Waddington, and apparently should have had their landing gear down to indicate that they were friendly aircraft passing through the airspace controlled by another group. Accompanying Hampdens from the Waddington flight landed at Drem, and the atmosphere in the mess that night was rather frosty!

UNKNOWN - Pre 1952

Wreck No :	88	Date Sunk :	Pre-1952
Latitude :	56 00 10 N	Longitude :	03 09 40 W
Decca Lat :	5600.17 N	Decca Long :	0309.67 W
Location :	near Leith Docks entrance	Area :	Leith
Type :		Tonnage :	
Length : feet	Beam : feet	Draught :	feet
How Sunk :		Depth :	6 metres

An unknown obstruction which may be a wreck or a rock, was reported by the receiver of wrecks at Leith in 1952. Could this be the *Bayonet*? This position is slightly to the South of one of the three anchorage points charted as L5, about one mile North of Leith docks.

There is a report of a submarine conning tower having been found within the swing clearance circle of one of these anchorage points. The remainder of the submarine is said to be buried.

CHAPTER 4

THE WRECKS OF INCHKEITH, INCHCOLM & ROSYTH

INTRODUCTION

Inchkeith is 4 miles from Leith and 3 miles from Kinghorn. It is about a mile long, triangular in shape, and about $^1/_4$ mile across at its widest, northern end. The highest point, upon which the lighthouse was built in 1803-1804, is 180 feet above sea level. Long Craig Reef and Briggs Reef extend for a further mile towards the south of the island, which is surrounded, particularly towards the south and west by relatively shallow water. The island is now owned by Tom Farmer of Kwik-Fit.

Inchcolm, (the Island of St. Columba), is the most beautiful of all the islands in the Forth. The well-preserved ruins of its monastery, founded in 1123 AD by Alexander I, are worth a visit. The island has been called the *Iona of the East*.

Sir William Mortimer, a nobleman who had caused displeasure to the monks during his lifetime, had arranged for his body to be buried on Inchcolm. As his coffin was being shipped out to the island, however, it was dumped overboard into one of the deepest parts of the Forth, about $^3/_4$ mile from Inchcolm, and known to this day as *Mortimer's Deep*.

The dockyard at Rosyth has been a major base for the Royal Navy particularly in the two world wars. It is interesting to divers not least because it offers the only recompression facilities in the area. Port Edgar on the South side of the River opposite Rosyth (just up-river of the Forth Road Bridge) was a minesweeper base but has now been developed into a yacht marina offering very good launching facilities.

The eastern area of the Forth offers the greatest variety of launching possibilities, from the old ferry slips at South Queensferry and North Queensferry, Dalgety Bay, Kinghorn and Burntisland.

One group of North Queensferry-based divers makes frequent dive trips in their Searider, from North Queensferry to the May Island, about 40 miles away! (Actions speak louder than words, which is suggestive of their opinion about launching facilities on the Forth !)

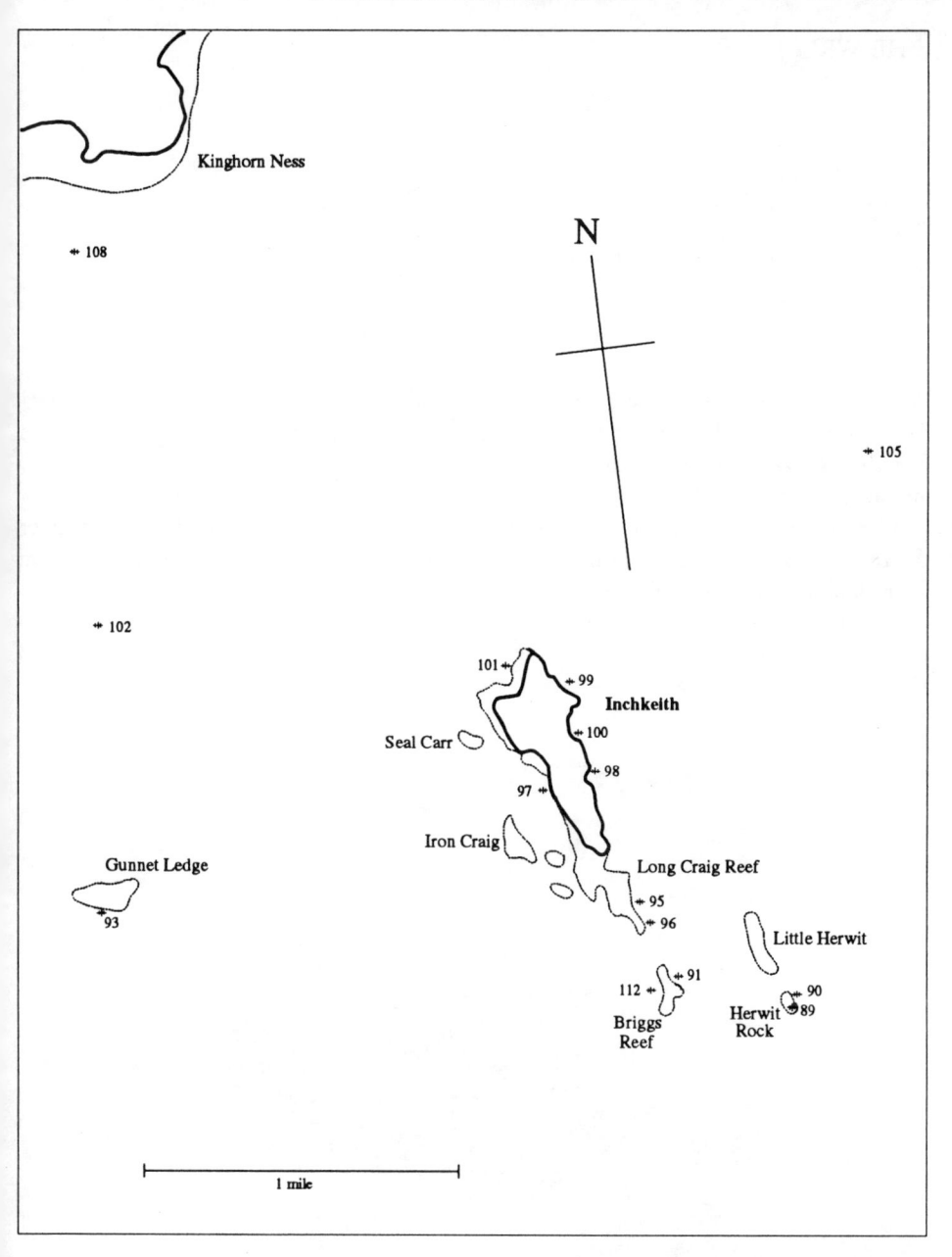

Chart showing the location of wrecks lying between Kinghorn Ness and the island of Inchkeith. The concentration in the vicinity of Inchkeith is apparent.

THE WRECKS

SWITHA

Wreck No :	89	Date Sunk :	31 01 1980
Latitude :	56 01 11 N	Longitude :	03 06 38 W
Decca Lat :	5601.18 N	Decca Long :	0306.63 W
Location :	Herwit Rock, S. of Inchkeith	Area :	Inchkeith
Type :	Fisheries Patrol	Tonnage :	573 gross
Length :	178.0 feet Beam : 30.0 feet	Draught :	15.0 feet
How Sunk :	Ran aground	Depth :	metres

Despite radio warnings that she was running into danger, HM Fisheries Protection vessel *Switha*, (ex-*Earnest Holt*), built in 1948 by Cochrane & Sons of Selby, ran aground on the Herwit Rock about a mile South of Inchkeith, in rough seas and gale Force winds at 4.40 am on 31st January 1980.

The Anstruther lifeboat took over two hours in the prevailing stormy conditions to cover the 18 miles to the wreck. All 25 aboard were airlifted to safety by a Sea King helicopter from RAF Boulmer in Northumberland.

Attempts to refloat her were unsuccessful, and on 7th February explosives were used to release her remaining fuel oil "to avoid further pollution". The wreck remained perched on Herwit Rock, and her back was soon broken by wave action.

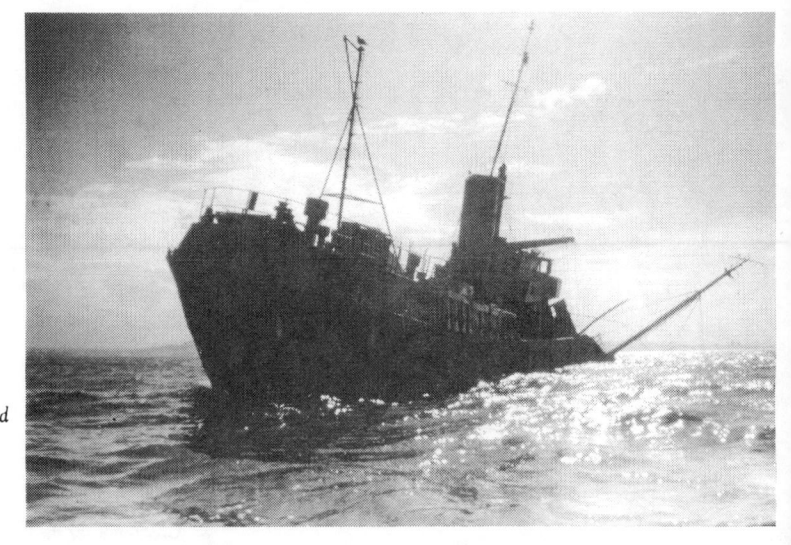

The Switha, wrecked on Herwit Rock (photograph by

She is now almost completely broken in two, but still prominently visible above water at all states of the tide. Storms over the years have gradually taken their toll, particularly one

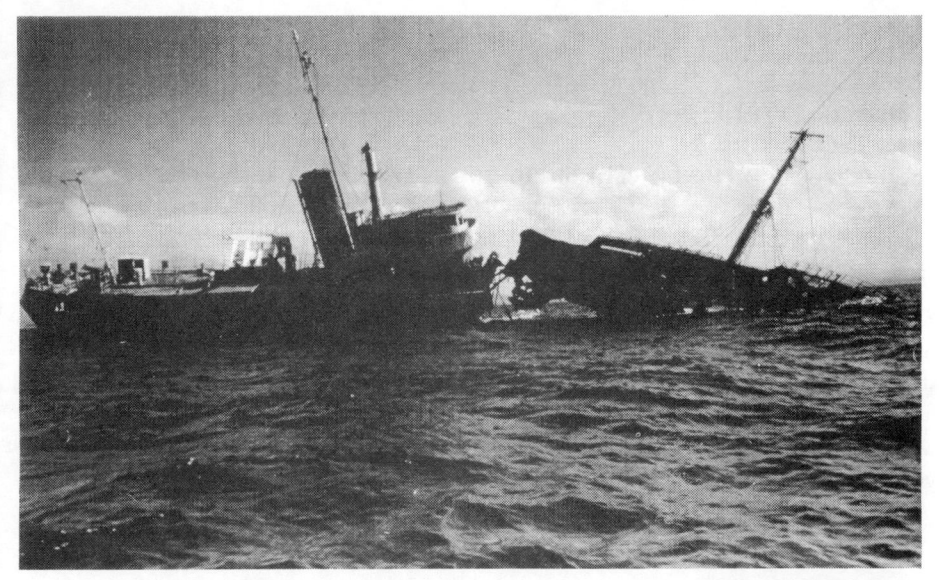

The Switha (photograph by Bob Baird)

in early January 1992, which significantly widened the gap between the bow section, which is lying on its starboard side, and the remainder of the wreck which is upright, but with a slight list to starboard. As might be expected, all non-ferrous items are long gone.

DEERHOUND ?

Wreck No :	90	Date Sunk :	25 03 1885
Latitude :	56 01 12 N	Longitude :	03 06 38 W
Decca Lat :	5601.20 N	Decca Long :	0306.63 W
Location :	Herwit Rock, S of Inchkeith	Area :	Inchkeith
Type :	Trawler	Tonnage :	20 gross
Length :	feet Beam : feet	Draught :	feet
How Sunk :	Ran aground	Depth :	5 metres

The Leith-registered iron-hulled steam trawler *Deerhound* was lost at Inchkeith on 25th March 1885.

This wreck was first reported in 1920, and there must be some doubt about her being the steam trawler *Deerhound*, as the wreck is of a considerably larger vessel than one of only 20 tons.

She lies very broken up, with her bows pointing North, and her stern very close to the starboard side of the *Switha*. Her boiler lies a few yards to the South, off the port side of the *Switha*, and breaks the surface at low water springs.

VIGILANT

Wreck No :	91	Date Sunk :	28 12 1882
Latitude :	56 01 15 N PA	Longitude :	03 07 18 W PA
Decca Lat :	5601.25 N	Decca Long :	0307.30 W
Location :	Briggs Reef, S of Inchkeith	Area :	Inchkeith
Type :	Brig	Tonnage :	303 gross
Length :	125.4 feet Beam : 25.4 feet	Draught :	14.9 feet
How Sunk :	Ran aground	Depth :	metres

Shortly after leaving Wemyss for Christiania on 28th December 1882, the 3-masted 247 ton net Norwegian brig *Vigilant* was wrecked on Briggs Reef, South of Inchkeith in a W by N storm.

It seems a curious action on the part of her master to choose to set out in such severe weather conditions. The phrase "any port in a storm" cannot have meant much to him. The voyage came to an abrupt end after only about 7 miles!

Wreckage from this schooner will most likely be at the West side of Briggs Reef.

RUNSWICK ?

Wreck No :	92	Date Sunk :	29 07 1889
Latitude :	56 01 17 N	Longitude :	03 04 42 W
Decca Lat :	5601.28 N	Decca Long :	0304.70 W
Location :	1 mile E of Herwit Rock	Area :	Inchkeith
Type :	Steamship	Tonnage :	324 gross
Length :	145.2 feet Beam : 26.4 feet	Draught :	13.2 feet
How Sunk :	Ran aground	Depth :	6 metres

A foul at 5.9 metres is charted in the above position, and in 1966, a wreck was reported to be standing up 4 metres from the bottom in a total depth of 10 metres. This would seem to suggest that the wreck may be more intact than one would expect of a vessel in such shallow water - perhaps sheltered to some extent by the reef..

This may possibly be the *Runswick*, an iron steamship of 324 tons gross, which stranded on Craigmore (Craigwaugh ?) rocks on 29 July 1889. On the other hand, I have come across a reference to the 197 ton trawler *Ben Gulvain* having been mined while on Admiralty service on 27 December 1940 at 560112N 030500W, extremely close to the above position. Curiously, this vessel is not mentioned in *British Vessels Lost at Sea, 1939-45* as either having been sunk or damaged.

POSSIBLE TRANSITS:
1) *Switha* in line with Inchmickery.
2) Grain elevator at Leith in line with Edinburgh Castle.
3) 40° to Narrow Deep red navigation buoy.
4) 320° to North Craig green navigation buoy.

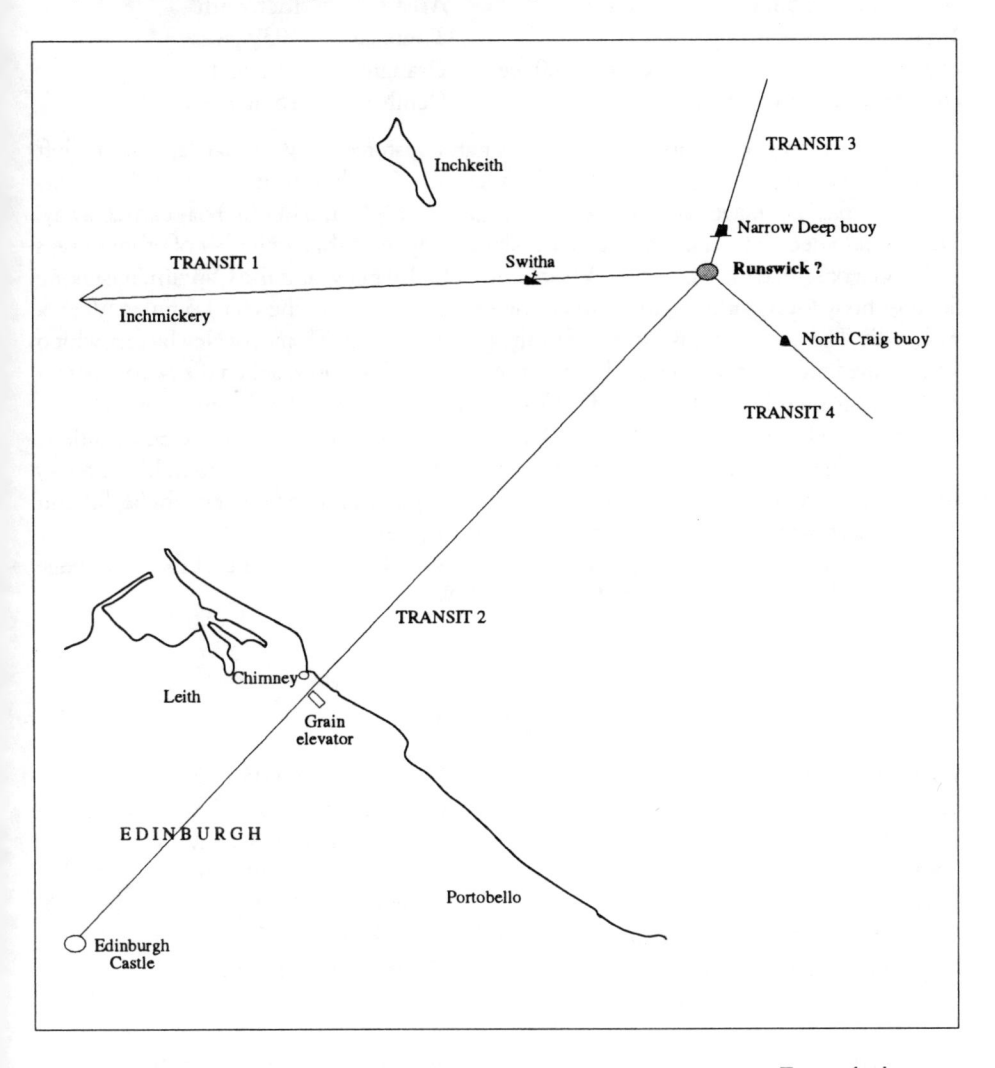

Transits for the Runswick, lost in 1889 near Herwit Rock

PAOLO

Wreck No :	93	Date Sunk :	19 10 1898
Latitude :	56 01 24 N PA	Longitude :	03 10 30 W PA
Decca Lat :	5601.40 N	Decca Long :	0311.00 W
Location :	1.5 miles W of Inchkeith	Area :	Inchkeith
Type :	Steamship	Tonnage :	1039 gross
Length :	224.4 feet Beam : 33.0 feet	Draught :	13.2 feet
How Sunk :	Ran aground	Depth :	16 metres

The *Paolo* was an iron steamship of 647 tons net, registered in West Hartlepool. She left Burntisland for Hamburg on Saturday 15th October 1898, but in the vicinity of the May Island was badly damaged in a severe Easterly gale, Force 9, and her lifeboat carried away. The Captain decided to put back to Burntisland. It appears that a number of other vessels in the area obscured his view of the West Gunnet Ledge buoy, and the Captain, mistaking the East buoy for it, sailed right between the two and struck on the reef 1.5 miles West of Inchkeith. The accident was witnessed by the pilot boat *Mary Thomas* of Newhaven, which went immediately to the rescue. The last of the 18 crew had just reached the *Mary Thomas* when the steamer lurched back and sank in 3 fathoms of water, becoming a total loss.

Gunnet Ledge is at 560124N, 031030W. An anchor chain runs from the South side of Gunnet Ledge and disappears into the mud, but the wreck has not been found. The rocky area is not too large to search, although if she has completely broken up, it might be difficult to distinguish wreckage from rock with an echo sounder.

The 20 ton drifter *Persevere* was mined 75 yards, 074 degrees from East Gunnet Ledge Buoy on 27th October 1940. (560122N, 031024W).

SAPPHO

Wreck No :	94	Date Sunk :	05 03 1900
Latitude :	56 01 26 N	Longitude :	03 04 20 W
Decca Lat :	5601.43 N	Decca Long :	0304.33 W
Location :	Craig Rocks	Area :	Inchkeith
Type :	Steamship	Tonnage :	1275 gross
Length :	231.0 feet Beam : 33.0 feet	Draught :	16.5 feet
How Sunk :	Ran aground	Depth :	11 metres

This was reported in 1966 to be a fairly large wreck standing up 4 metres in 10 metres.

Sappho, 1275 tons gross, 70 x 10 x 5m, (i.e. 231 x 33 x 16.5 feet), stranded on Craigwaugh Rocks in March 1900.

POSSIBLE TRANSITS:
1) Narrow Deep buoy in line with the radio mast above Burntisland.
2) 130° 200 metres from Narrow Deep red navigation buoy. (50° to the red buoy).
3) 100° to the red and white South Channel approach buoy.

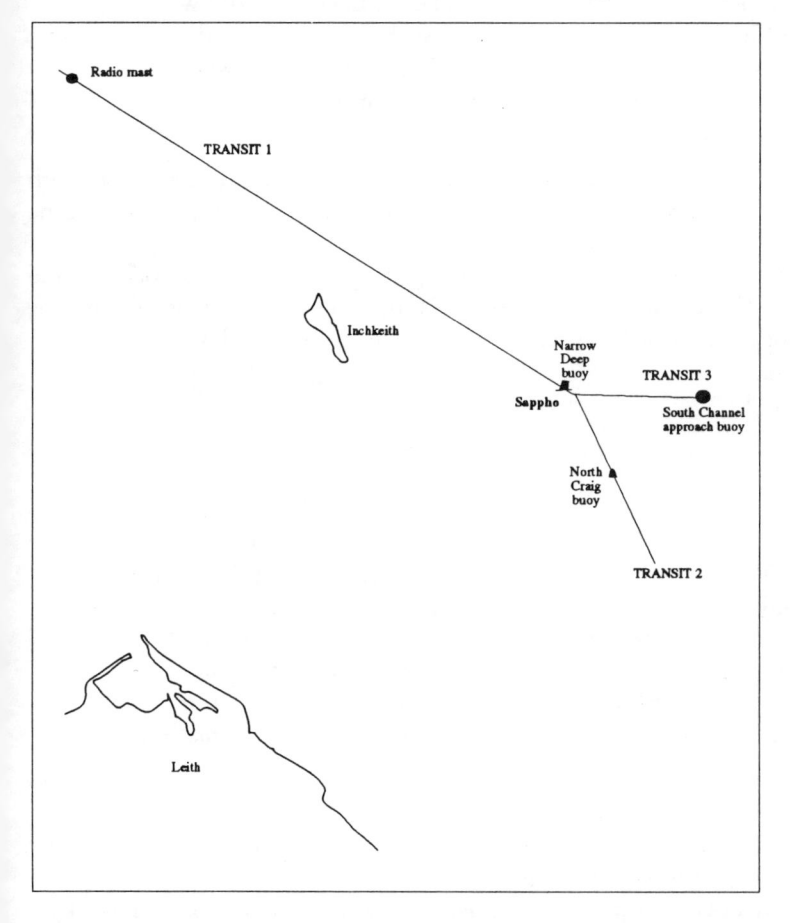

Transits for the Sappho, lost in 1900 near Craig Rocks

Before setting off on her maiden voyage from Burntisland to Rotterdam with a cargo of coal, the British Steam Navigation Company's new steamship *Sappho*, built by Ramage and Ferguson of Leith, ran her trial entirely satisfactorily during the afternoon of Monday 5th March 1900. At 7 pm the party of guests on board were transferred to another vessel in Leith Roads, and the *Sappho* then proceeded on her voyage in clear weather and a calm sea. About an hour later she ran on to South Craig Rocks at 11 knots. It was soon realised that the vessel was in a dangerous position, and the 16 crew collected their belongings, left the steamer, which was lying bow down at low water, and landed at Leith. It was feared that she would break in two and become a total wreck. In an attempt to save the vessel, deck fittings were stripped off, but within a few days, the *Sappho* settled stern first on the bottom.

ANNIE COWLEY

Wreck No :	95	Date Sunk :	09 01 1890
Latitude :	56 01 30 N PA	Longitude :	03 08 00 W PA
Decca Lat :	5601.50 N	Decca Long :	0308.00 W
Location :	Inchkeith	Area :	Inchkeith
Type :	Schooner	Tonnage :	64 gross
Length :	feet Beam : feet	Draught :	feet
How Sunk :	Ran aground	Depth :	metres

The 64 ton wooden schooner *Annie Cowley* stranded at Inchkeith while en route from Leith to Crail in ballast on 9th January 1890. A Westerly severe gale, Force 9 was blowing at the time.

The position 560130N, 030800W is only a rough estimate. Because of the wind direction, she would have struck on the West side of Inchkeith, or more probably on Long Craig Reef, or Briggs Reef which extend for a mile South of the island.

GHIDO

Wreck No :	96	Date Sunk :	21 12 1900
Latitude :	56 01 30 N PA	Longitude :	03 08 00 W PA
Decca Lat :	5601.50 N	Decca Long :	0308.00 W
Location :	Rocks S of Inchkeith	Area :	Inchkeith
Type :	Schooner	Tonnage :	159 gross
Length :	feet Beam : feet	Draught :	feet
How Sunk :	Ran aground	Depth :	metres

The Russian schooner *Ghido*, en route from St. Davids to Rye, was blown on to the rocks South of Inchkeith in a Westerly storm on 21st December 1900.

The reefs running to the South of Inchkeith extend Southward for a mile, and she could be on either the Long Craig reef or Briggs reef.

These reefs have obviously claimed a number of vessels, as there is broken wreckage scattered along these reefs, which are also good for lobsters.

OSCAR DEN II

Wreck No :	97	Date Sunk :	16 11 1888
Latitude :	56 01 45 N PA	Longitude :	03 08 00 W PA
Decca Lat :	5601.75 N	Decca Long :	0308.00 W
Location :	Inchkeith	Area :	Inchkeith
Type :	Barque	Tonnage :	520 gross
Length : feet	Beam : feet	Draught :	feet
How Sunk :	Ran aground	Depth :	metres

The Norwegian barque *Oscar Den II* was en route from Sundswall to London with a cargo of firewood when she encountered a Force 10 SW storm. Progress directly into the gales must have been almost impossible, and she probably entered the Forth to seek shelter until the storm abated, but was blown on to Inchkeith and wrecked.

Because of the wind direction, she will likely be somewhere off the West side of the island itself, which is about a mile long, or along the reef which stretches a further mile out to sea, South of the island. No lives were reported lost, and in the sea conditions which were prevailing at the time, this suggests she may be more likely to be off the island itself, rather than the reef, as the crew may have survived by being washed ashore on the island, whereas if the vessel had hit the submerged reef, there would have been little possibility of the crew surviving.

GRIMSEL

Wreck No :	98	Date Sunk :	12 10 1889
Latitude :	56 01 54 N	Longitude :	03 07 48 W
Decca Lat :	5601.90 N	Decca Long :	0307.80 W
Location :	E side of Inchkeith	Area :	Inchkeith
Type :	Steamship	Tonnage :	1398 gross
Length : 251.0 feet	Beam : 34.2 feet	Draught :	17.5 feet
How Sunk :	Ran aground in fog	Depth :	4 metres

Grimsel was a British steamship built in 1880 by J. Redhead & Co.

En route from Salonica to Leith with a cargo of rye and five passengers, she ran aground in thick fog on the East side of Inchkeith.

The broken remains of the keel from the bows to the bridge lie covered in kelp in shallow water close to the shore at 560154N, 030748W. Brass bell dolphins 1 metre long have been recovered, along with the bell clapper, but the diver who recovered them in 1990 could find no trace of the bell itself. The stern section with the engine and boiler must lie slightly further out down the slope, but still in fairly shallow water.

SUNBEAM 1

Wreck No :	99		Date Sunk :	16 04 1918
Latitude :	56 02 00 N PA		Longitude :	03 08 00 W PA
Decca Lat :	5602.00 N		Decca Long :	0308.00 W
Location :	Inchkeith		Area :	Inchkeith
Type :	Drifter		Tonnage :	133 gross
Length :	100.0 feet	Beam : 20.1 feet	Draught :	10.1 feet
How Sunk :	Collision		Depth :	metres

Sunbeam 1 was a 75 ton drifter employed as an examination vessel, which sank after a collision at Inchkeith on 16th April 1918. (With what?)

Sunbeam - iron screw ketch (steam trawler) 133 tons gross, 100.0 x 20.1 x 10.1 feet built by Hawthorns & Co., Leith in 1891 and registered in Dundee, appears in the 1916-17 edition of *Lloyds Register of Shipping*. (She was 49 tons net).

Sunbeam 1 - a 75 ton drifter, does not appear in that edition of the register. (Does it appear in the 1917-18 edition?).

LUCIE

Wreck No :	100		Date Sunk :	28 03 1898
Latitude :	56 02 00 N PA		Longitude :	03 08 00 W PA
Decca Lat :	5602.00 N		Decca Long :	0308.00 W
Location :	E side of Inchkeith		Area :	Inchkeith
Type :	Brig		Tonnage :	203 gross
Length :	feet	Beam : feet	Draught :	feet
How Sunk :	Ran aground		Depth :	metres

The Swedish brig *Lucie*, with a cargo of pit props from Gothenburg to Bo'ness, was blown ashore on Inchkeith by a North-easterly severe gale, Force 9, on 28th March 1898.

That suggests her remains will be somewhere along the East side of Inchkeith.

PAUL

Wreck No :	101		Date Sunk :	16 11 1888
Latitude :	56 02 00 N PA		Longitude :	03 08 00 W PA
Decca Lat :	5602.00 N		Decca Long :	0308.00 W
Location :	Inchkeith		Area :	Inchkeith
Type :	Brig		Tonnage :	135 gross

Length :	feet	Beam :	feet
How Sunk :	Ran aground		
Draught :	feet		
Depth :	metres		

The 135 ton German brig *Paul*, en route from Bremerhaven to West Wemyss, was blown on to Inchkeith in a WSW storm on 16th November 1888. Because of the wind direction, I should imagine she must lie at the West side of Inchkeith.

SAUCY

Wreck No :	102	Date Sunk :	04 09 1940
Latitude :	56 02 10 N	Longitude :	03 10 33 W
Decca Lat :	5602.17 N	Decca Long :	0310.55 W
Location :	1.25 miles WNW of Inchkeith	Area :	Inchkeith
Type :	Tug	Tonnage :	579 gross
Length :	155.3 feet Beam : 31.1 feet	Draught :	15.7 feet
How Sunk :	Mined	Depth :	13 metres

The *Saucy* was a 579 ton steel tug built in 1918 by Livingston & Cooper of Hessle. There were some casualties when she was mined at 19.35 hrs on 4th September 1940.

The Navy looked for her in 1967 but did not find her, and considered that she may be silted over. Perhaps they were simply looking in the wrong position!

INTEGRITY ?

Wreck No :	103	Date Sunk :	07 10 1879
Latitude :	56 02 16 N	Longitude :	03 11 48 W
Decca Lat :	5602.27 N	Decca Long :	0311.80 W
Location :	1.5 miles SE of Burntisland	Area :	Inchkeith
Type :	Trawler	Tonnage :	
Length :	feet Beam : feet	Draught :	feet
How Sunk :	Collision	Depth :	31 metres

In thick fog, the steam trawler *Integrity* sank in five minutes after being in collision with the 427 ton iron paddle steamer *John Stirling*, which was on her usual route from Granton to Burntisland. The trawler's crew of seven were picked up and taken to Burntisland by the *John Stirling*. Compensation of £870 plus costs was made by the North British Railway Co. who owned the *John Stirling*.

The *Integrity* must lie somewhere along the ferry route. The only *Unknown* I am aware of reasonably close to that route is the wreck charted at 520616N, 031148W, 1.5 miles South East of Burntisland.

CAMPANIA

Wreck No :	104	Date Sunk :	05 11 1918
Latitude :	56 02 26 N	Longitude :	03 13 20 W
Decca Lat :	5602.43 N	Decca Long :	0313.33 W
Location :	1 mile S of Burntisland	Area :	Inchkeith
Type :	Aircraft carrier	Tonnage :	18000 gross
Length :	622.0 feet Beam : 65.2 feet	Draught :	37.8 feet
How Sunk :	Collision with *Royal Oak*	Depth :	27 metres

The 18000 ton Cunard liner *Campania*, measuring 622 x 65.2 x 37.8 feet was built by Fairfields in 1893, but was converted into an aircraft carrier during the first world war.

After the end of that war she was moored off Burntisland with a number of other Royal Navy ships. During a storm on 5th November 1918 her anchor chain snapped. and she drifted into several of the other ships, including the battleships *Royal Oak* and *Glorious*, but the fatal damage was inflicted by her collision with the forefoot of the battleship HMS *Revenge*, as a result of which she sank quickly by the stern. All her crew were saved.

This wreck is of such a size that for a time after she sank, she was a hazard to navigation until she was dispersed to give a clearance of 6.5 fathoms (12 metres) in 1947.

The wreck is in two parts close together about 1 mile South of Burntisland Harbour. The positions are 560226N, 031320W and 560220N, 031324W. She lies on a muddy bottom, and underwater visibility in this area is usually very bad, making it difficult to know which part of the wreck you are on.

Extensive salvage was carried out in the late 1960s, suggesting that there must be times when the visibility is sufficiently good to allow this.

This is the largest ship sunk in the Forth, and despite the salvage, a vessel of this size must still be worth a visit.

On pages 82-83 : *Dramatic images of the end of a warship - the HMS Campania sinking*

Top left : A plane's searchlight illuminates the Campania before dawn as she begins to settle on the 5th November 1918.

Middle left : The scene shortly after dawn at 8.00 am as the Capania settles by the stern.

Bottom left : By 8.20 am the vessel is listing to port as she settles further.

Top right : The list has increased substantially by 8.30 am

Middle right : The vessel is well heeled over and almost on the bottom by 8.40 am

Bottom right : The Campania at 8.50 am having settled on the seabed with her masts and funnels standing clear of the water.

All photographs show the port side of the vessel, except the first which shows the starboard.

(All photographs courtesy of Conway Picture Library)

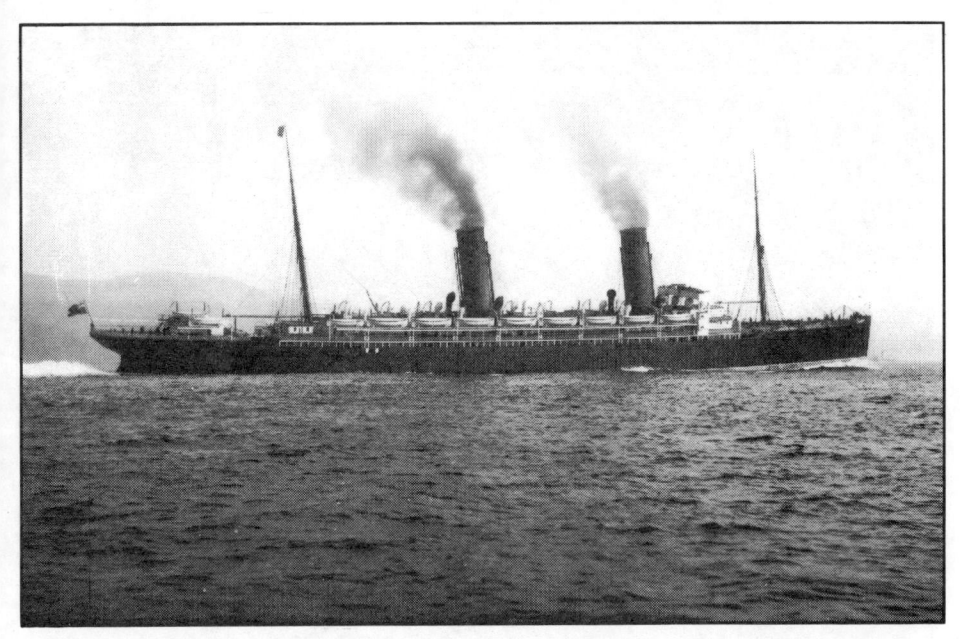

Below: The Campania as a Royal Navy aircraft carrier, lost in 1918, when she drifted on to the warships Royal Oak, Glorious and Revenge. (Photograph courtesy of Imperial War Museum).

Above: The record-breaking Cunard passenger liner Campania, built in 1893, at the Princes Landing Stage, Liverpool. (Photograph reproduced with the permission of Glasgow University Archives).

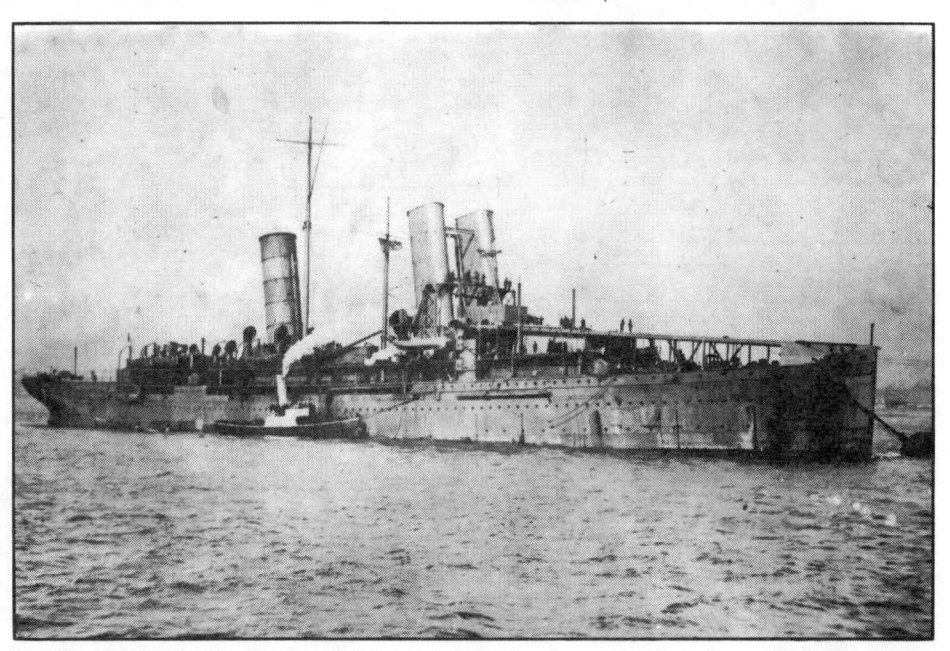

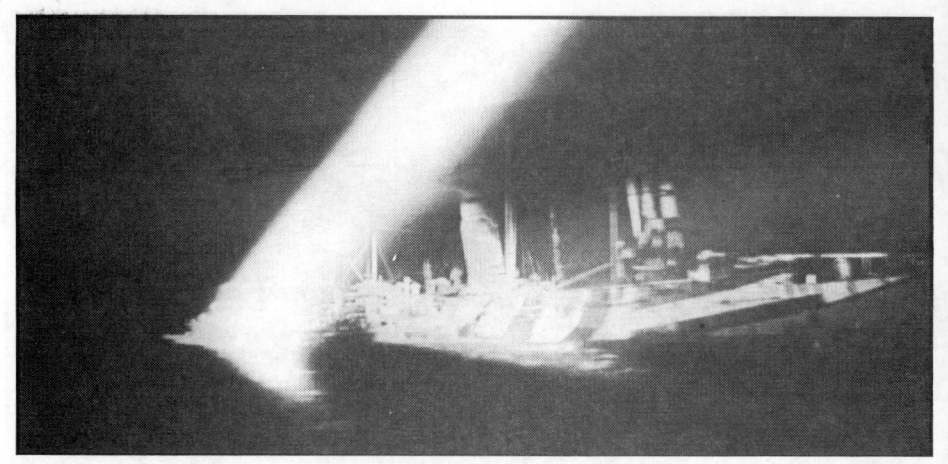

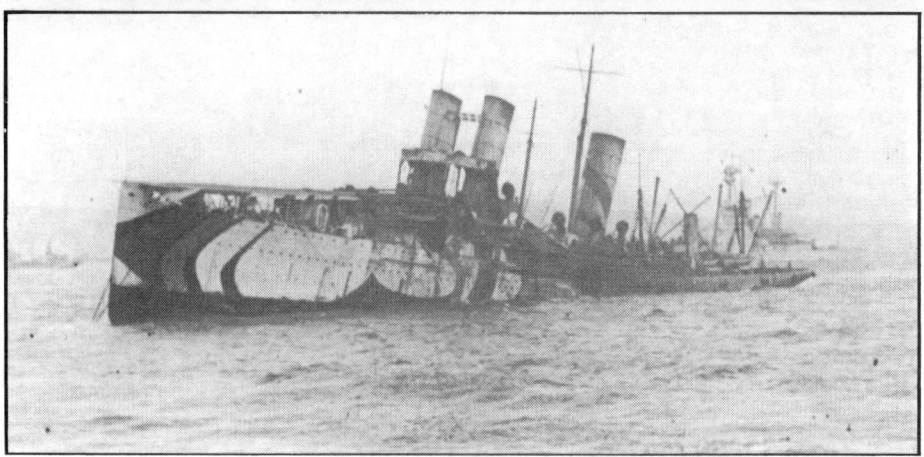

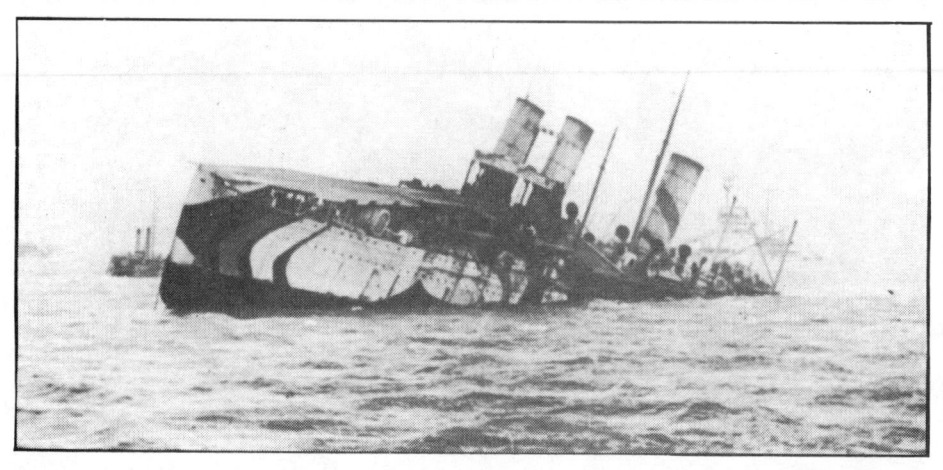

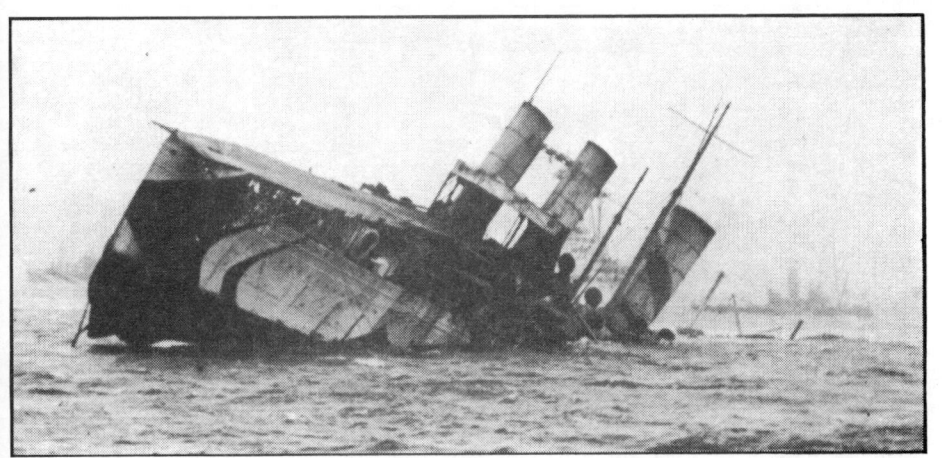

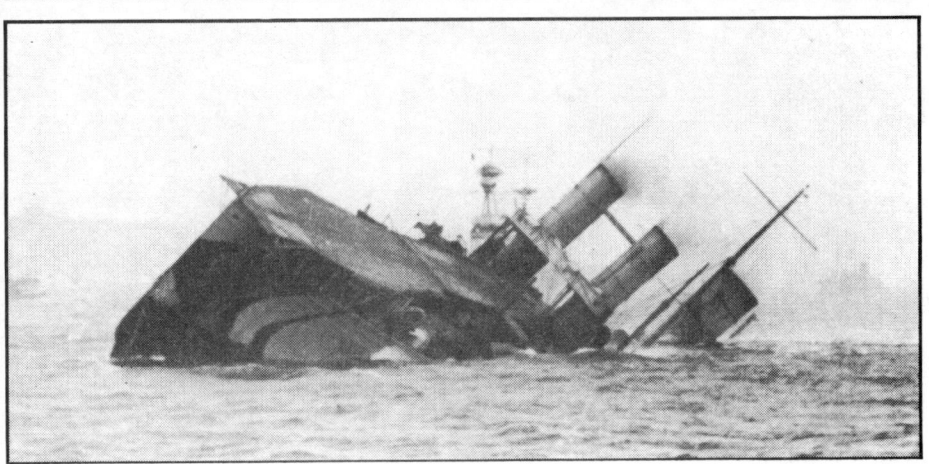

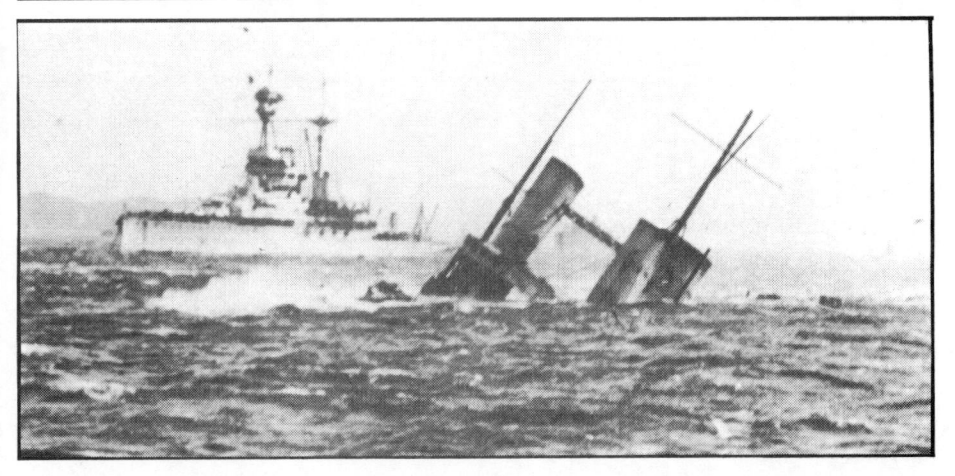

Inchkeith, Inchcolm & Rosyth

Location of the Campania

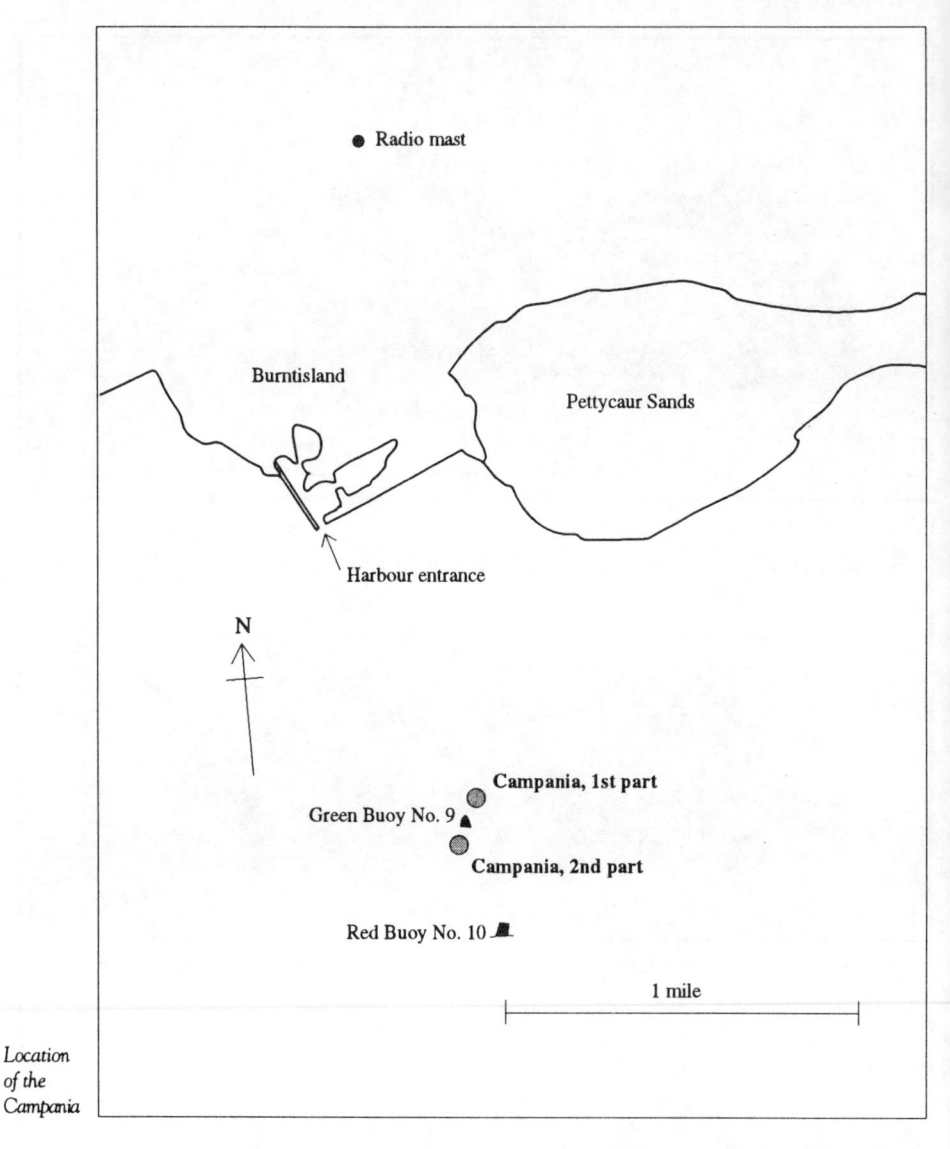

The two parts of the ship lie close to the green navigation buoy No. 9, one mile directly out from the entrance to Burntisland harbour, and rise up about 15 metres from the bottom.

Each part is only about 150 yards from the buoy, one to the NNE (20° magnetic to the buoy), the other to the SSW (200° magnetic to the buoy). They can be easily found by echo sounding around the buoy.

GOOD DESIGN

Wreck No :	105	**Date Sunk :**	23 11 1940
Latitude :	56 02 56 N	**Longitude :**	03 06 20 W
Decca Lat :	5602.93 N	**Decca Long :**	0306.33 W
Location :	1.25 miles NE of Inchkeith	**Area :**	Inchkeith
Type :	HM motor patrol	**Tonnage :**	46 gross
Length :	72.0 feet **Beam :** 15.0 feet	**Draught :**	4.5 feet
How Sunk :	Mined, towed Granton	**Depth :**	25 metres

Six hundred HDMLs were built between 1940-1944. They had two diesel engines, Gardner, Gleniffer or Thorneycroft, and were armed with two 20 mm guns.

Two of the six crew of the *Good Design* were killed when the vessel struck a mine, and broke in two.

It was not until after I had spent a considerable time abortively looking for the wreck, that I discovered the two halves were towed to Granton.

There are extremely strong tidal streams in this area - far stronger than the chart suggests!

SNOWDROP

Wreck No :	106	**Date Sunk :**	13 02 1869
Latitude :	56 03 20 N PA	**Longitude :**	03 05 12 W PA
Decca Lat :	5603.33 N	**Decca Long :**	0305.20 W
Location :	2 miles ENE of Inchkeith	**Area :**	Inchkeith
Type :	Schooner	**Tonnage :**	141 gross
Length :	feet **Beam :** feet	**Draught :**	feet
How Sunk :	Collision	**Depth :**	metres

While inward-bound for Leith on 13th February 1869 with a cargo of peas, beans and tares (a legume of the same family as peas and beans, used as animal food) from Pillau, the 141 ton Aberdeen schooner *Snowdrop* was involved in a collision with a vessel bound for Wemyss. She was taken in tow by the Leith steam tug *Pet* and, as they proceeded up the Forth, the wind gradually increased in violence to a storm. At about 5.00 pm the storm compelled the captain of the *Pet* to cast the schooner adrift for his own vessel's safety, particularly as he was by then running short of coal. When the *Pet* left, the *Snowdrop* anchored and endeavoured to ride out the storm, which increased in intensity, with a heavy sea. Although another vessel in the vicinity observed that the schooner was in great distress, no assistance could be rendered.

The *Snowdrop*'s lights were seen until about 7.00 pm, about which time it is supposed that she foundered with the loss of all six of the crew. The tops of her masts could be seen at low water the next day, 2 miles ENE of Inchkeith, and a boat belonging to the *Snowdrop* was found adrift in the Forth and taken to Crail.

GOODWILL

Wreck No :	107	Date Sunk :	02 11 1940
Latitude :	56 03 28 N PA	Longitude :	03 03 00 W PA
Decca Lat :	5603.47 N	Decca Long :	0303.00 W
Location :	3.1 miles 073° from Inchkeith	Area :	Inchkeith
Type :	Drifter	Tonnage :	
Length :	feet Beam : feet	Draught :	feet
How Sunk :	Mined	Depth :	23 metres

The patrol drifter *Goodwill* struck a mine and sank 073° 3.1 miles from Inchkeith at 11.55 hrs on 2nd November 1940.

It would seem that she strayed a little too far North of the swept channel, into part of the defensive minefield.

HEIMA

Wreck No :	108	Date Sunk :	15 03 1905
Latitude :	56 03 30 N PA	Longitude :	03 11 00 W PA
Decca Lat :	5603.50 N	Decca Long :	0311.00 W
Location :	Off Kinghorn	Area :	Inchkeith
Type :	Schooner	Tonnage :	
Length :	feet Beam : feet	Draught :	feet
How Sunk :	Ran aground	Depth :	metres

On 15th March 1905, the Norwegian schooner *Heima*, bound for Alloa with pit props, passed Kinghorn Ness, but owing to the terrific gale she missed stays and could not work round, with the result that she came ashore on the sand bank. The seven crew took to their boat, but it had hardly got clear when it was swamped, and the whole of the crew were thrown into the water. Fortunately all were wearing lifejackets, and were helped ashore by a number of artillery men belonging to the Kinghorn battery. Tugs were unable to refloat the vessel.

BOY ANDREW

Wreck No :	109	Date Sunk :	09 11 1941
Latitude :	56 03 31 N	Longitude :	03 01 55 W
Decca Lat :	5603.52 N	Decca Long :	0301.92 W
Location :	5 miles SW of Kirkcaldy	Area :	Inchkeith
Type :	Drifter	Tonnage :	97 gross
Length :	feet Beam : feet	Draught :	feet
How Sunk :	Collision with *St. Rognvald*	Depth :	27 metres

This wreck is known to local fishermen as the *Mussels Wreck*, and is very close to the approximate position given for the sinking of the *Boy Andrew* in 1941 (560342N, 030136W PA). It could not be found during a search around that PA in 1960. It is charted (Chart 735, Aug. 1976), at 560320N, 030104W.

Boy Andrew (ex-*Sunburst*), was an Admiralty drifter built in 1918, and requisitioned in 1940 for use as an auxiliary patrol vessel.

On the morning of 9th November 1941 the steamship *St. Rognvald* was overtaking the *Boy Andrew* in a swept channel when the drifter suddenly went to starboard across the course of the *St. Rognvald*. The drifter was pushed bodily under water and all her crew of 13 were drowned. The court of enquiry took the view that the *St. Rognvald*'s course was too close to the *Boy Andrew*, and that this was not good seamanship. She could have given the *Boy Andrew* a wider clearance, but both vessels, by faulty navigation, contributed to the disaster, the apportionment of blame being two thirds to the *Boy Andrew* and one third to the *St. Rognvald*. This decision was upheld by a court of appeal in 1947.

While searching for this wreck in 1990, we manoeuvred alongside a fishing boat trawling very close to this position. The trawler skipper pointed out the wreck position a short distance off his course, and we dropped a shot line on the wreck when it appeared on our echo sounder. While kitting up and waiting for the trawl net to pass safely before putting divers in the water, however, our shot line was caught in the trawl and swept away!

MORAL: Beware of trawlers! Their nets can extend an awfully long way behind the vessel.

IRIS

Wreck No :	110	Date Sunk :	27 04 1912
Latitude :	56 04 00 N PA	Longitude :	03 04 00 W PA
Decca Lat :	5604.00 N	Decca Long :	0304.00 W
Location :	5 miles E by N of Inchkeith	Area :	Inchkeith
Type :	Steamship	Tonnage :	149 gross
Length :	feet Beam : feet	Draught :	feet
How Sunk :	Collision with *Cayo Manzanillo*	Depth :	metres

The 149 ton Danish steamship *Iris* left Dysart on 27th April 1912, bound for Treguier, France, but was sunk in a collision with the London steamship *Cayo Manzanillo* 5 miles E by N of Inchkeith.

SALVESTRIA

Wreck No :	111	**Date Sunk :**	27 07 1940
Latitude :	56 04 03 N	**Longitude :**	03 04 07 W
Decca Lat :	5604.04 N	**Decca Long :**	0304.12 W
Location :	2.77 miles NE of Inchkeith Lt.	**Area :**	Inchkeith
Type :	Tanker	**Tonnage :**	11938 gross
Length :	500.3 feet **Beam :** 62.4 feet	**Draught :**	42.6 feet
How Sunk :	Mined	**Depth :**	27 metres

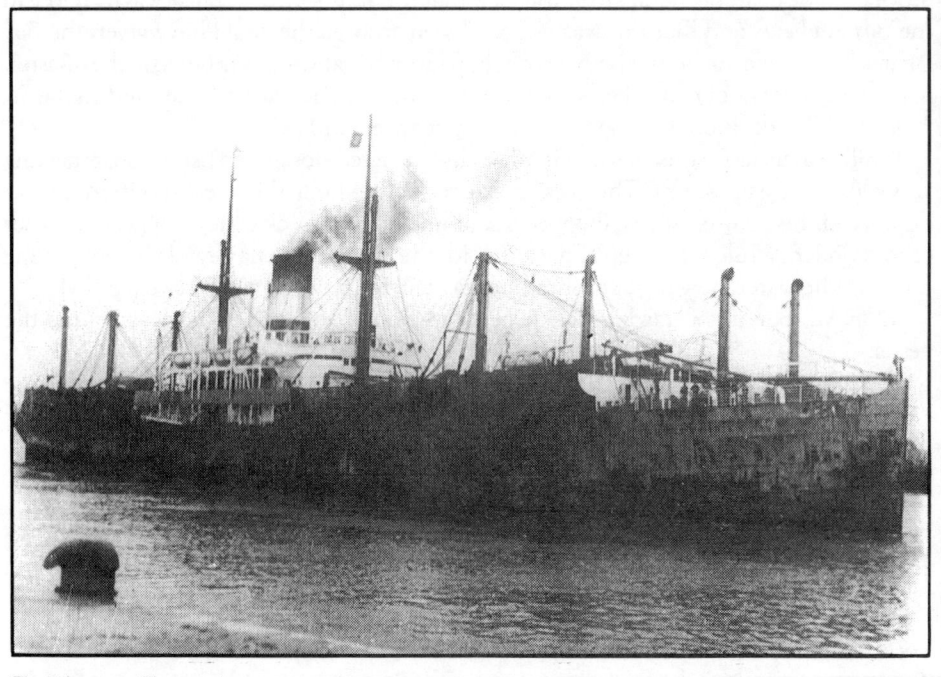

The Salvestria. (Photograph courtesy of Christian Salvesen).

The twin-screw steam engined tanker *Salvestria* (ex-*Cardiganshire*) was built in 1913 by Workman Clark of Belfast for the Royal Mail Steam Packet Co., and was converted in 1929 to a whaling factory ship for Christian Salvesen of Leith.

She was sunk by an acoustic mine when she strayed out of the swept channel while bringing fuel oil from Aruba to Rosyth, and was the first Salvesen ship to be sunk during the war. Ten of the crew of 57 were lost.

The wreck is charted as 14.4 metres. It may have been only 14.4 metres immediately after sinking, but salvage efforts have since reduced it to a large pile of scrap metal at 27 metres.

The highest point stands 5 metres off the sandy bottom and, as this wreck is very popular with sea anglers, there is lots of fishing tackle, grapnels, etc. entangled in the wreckage.

TRANSITS:
1) North tip of Inchkeith in line with centre of left hand gas holder at Granton.
2) Centre of three light-coloured blocks of flats in Kirkcaldy in line with West Lomond.
3) Fidra light open to right of Bass Rock by same distance as sea level to the top of Fidra light.
4) Chimneys at Cockenzie power station mid-way between red buoy No. 2 and green buoy No. 1.
5) Wreck of Switha in line with conspicuous chimney at Seafield, between Leith and Portobello.

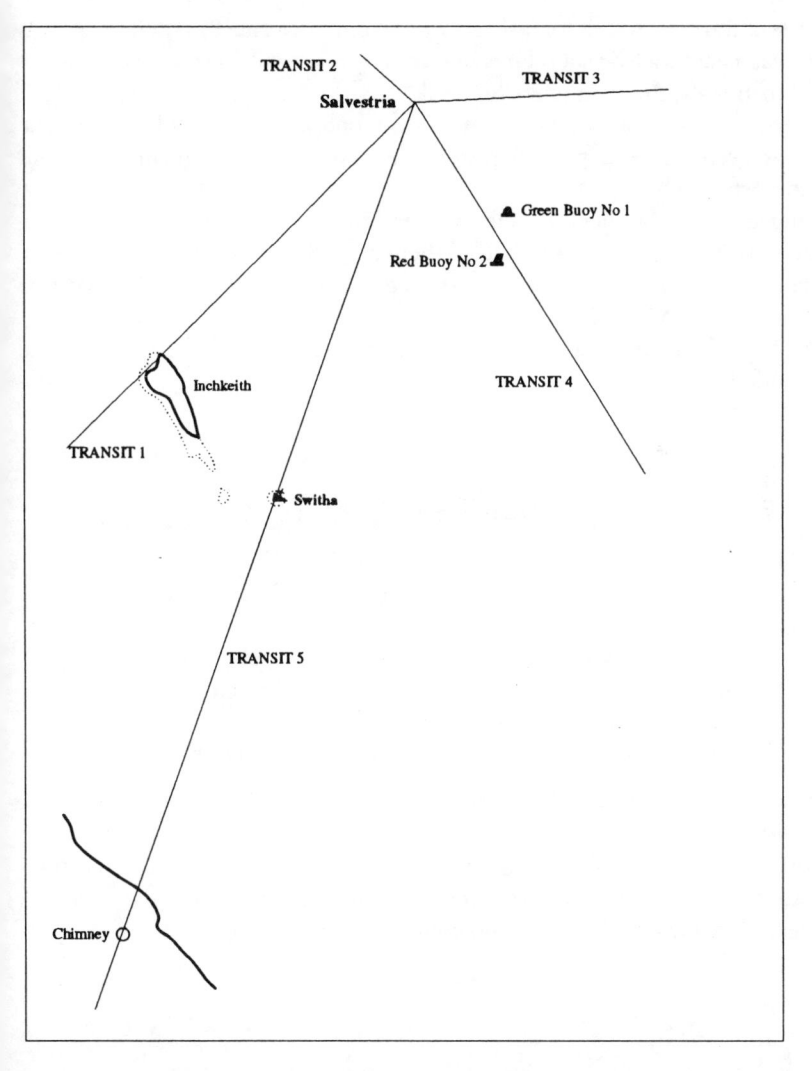

Sketch of the transits for the Salvestria

QUICKSTEP

Wreck No :	112	Date Sunk :	15 10 1907
Latitude :	56 01 12 N PA	Longitude :	03 07 24 W PA
Decca Lat :	5610.20 N	Decca Long :	0307.40 W
Location :	Briggs Reef, S of Inchkeith	Area :	Inchkeith
Type :	Steamship	Tonnage :	936 gross
Length :	210.3 feet Beam : 31.0 feet	Draught :	15.4 feet
How Sunk :	Ran aground	Depth :	metres

Shortly after leaving Leith on 15th October 1907 with a cargo of 1200 tons of coal for Rochester, the 588 tons net iron steamship *Quickstep* ran on to rocks South of Inchkeith.

All the efforts of the crew to call for assistance went unnoticed and, as their vessel was perched above water across a ledge of submerged rock, with about 2 metres depth of water forward and 10 metres aft, she soon broke her back.

Attempts were made to launch a boat, but it was found that this could not be done without incurring even greater danger than would be experienced by remaining aboard throughout the stormy night.

The following morning, the wreck was discovered by the tug *Transit*, which was visiting Inchkeith. She took off the 16 crew and landed them at Leith.

Although one report suggests the *Quickstep* ran on to Briggs Reef, could the *Quickstep* be the wreck adjacent to the *Switha* ?

The *Quickstep* was built in 1889 by J. Priestman, engined by North East Marine and registered in Sunderland.

ABERTAY?

Wreck No :	113	Date Sunk :	10 10 1892
Latitude :	56 00 57 N	Longitude :	03 21 12 W
Decca Lat :	5600.95 N	Decca Long :	0321.20 W
Location :	1 mile E of Carlingnose Point	Area :	Inchcolm
Type :	Steamship	Tonnage :	635 gross
Length :	feet Beam : feet	Draught :	feet
How Sunk :	Collision with *Iron Duke*	Depth :	18 metres

There may be two wrecks here, or perhaps one wreck in two parts, most likely sunk as the result of a collision.

The steel steamship *Abertay* looks a likely candidate for the wreck charted in this position as, on 10th October 1892, she was lost in a collision with the battleship *HMS Iron Duke* near the Forth bridge, while outward bound from Grangemouth to Rostock.

ALLIANCE ?

Wreck No :	114	Date Sunk :	22 03 1905
Latitude :	56 01 14 N	Longitude :	03 18 27 W
Decca Lat :	5601.23 N	Decca Long :	0318.45 W
Location :	0.75 miles SSW of Inchcolm	Area :	Inchcolm
Type :	Steamship	Tonnage :	326 gross
Length :	145.2 feet Beam : 23.1 feet	Draught :	9.9 feet
How Sunk :	Ran aground	Depth :	25 metres

This wreck was located in April 1967, lying N/S, 160 feet long, 263° 5940 feet from Oxcars Light, in the main shipping channel! (I have a reference to this being sunk pre-1915.)

The Aberdeen steamship *Alliance*, from Inverkeithing to London with a cargo of stones from Carlingnose quarry, went on the rocks close to Inchcolm when starting her voyage in foggy conditions on Wednesday night, 22nd March, 1905. The vessel sank and the crew landed on the island.

The *Alliance* was an iron screw steamship of 326 tons gross, 191 tons net, belonging to the North Eastern Shipping Co. of Aberdeen.

However, it is doubtful if this wreck is the *Alliance*, in view of her position in the deep water of the main shipping channel, $^3/_4$ mile SSW of Inchcolm. It would seem much more likely that this is the wreck of a vessel which either foundered, or sank in a collision. This wreck is also apparently 15 feet longer than the *Alliance*, which is more likely to be near the position of the *Porthcawl*, close to 560136N, 031836W, just off the West of Inchcolm.

There are extremely strong tidal streams here in silty water.

UNKNOWN - 3 BARGES

Wreck No :	115	Date Sunk :	1955
Latitude :	56 01 24 N	Longitude :	03 21 24 W
Decca Lat :	5601.40 N	Decca Long :	0321.40 W
Location :	1 mile E of Carlingnose	Area :	Inchcolm
Type :	3 barges	Tonnage :	
Length :	feet Beam : feet	Draught :	feet
How Sunk :		Depth :	5 metres

Three steel barges carrying concrete ballast were sunk in 1955, and were reported in 1967 to have least depths of 62 feet and 50 feet Their positions are 560124N, 032112W, 560124N, 032115W and 560124N, 032124W.

PORTHCAWL

Wreck No :	116	Date Sunk :	01 02 1926
Latitude :	56 01 36 N	Longitude :	03 18 36 W
Decca Lat :	5601.60 N	Decca Long :	0318.60 W
Location :	200-300 yards W of Inchcolm	Area :	Inchcolm
Type :	Steamship	Tonnage :	2481 gross
Length :	298.5 feet Beam : 44.0 feet	Draught :	21.2 feet
How Sunk :	Ran aground	Depth :	4 metres

Porthcawl was a steel screw steamship built at Burntisland in 1923, and registered in Cardiff. Her engine was made by D. Rowan & Co. of Glasgow.

According to the Scotsman newspaper, the *Porthcawl* went ashore on the West side of Inchcolm on 1st February 1926, shortly after leaving Grangemouth with a cargo of 4000 tons of coal for Genoa. On 4th February, despite continuous pumping, the ship was still firmly on the rocks with serious bottom damage, the sides showing signs of strain, and some of the deck plates buckled, although it was hoped to make an attempt to refloat her in a day or two. The following day, it was reported that her back was broken in front of the bridge, and salvage was abandoned. In addition to the 4000 tons of cargo coal, a further 380 tons of coal was in her bunkers.

A report in *The Fifeshire Advertiser* of 6/2/1926 appears to give a different position, as it states that "The *Porthcawl*, with a crew of 23, went aground during an unusually high spring tide, a little way from Oxcar Light, which lies about 200 yards West of Inchcolm." A glance at the chart reveals an obvious error in that report, as Oxcar Light in fact lies 0.6 nautical miles, (about 1200 yards) South East of Inchcolm!

She was discovered to be lying between two reefs with her bow high and dry, and her hull buckling with a severe list. In daylight she could be seen from the shore. Underwater visibility in this area around the Middens Reef is generally very poor - I'm tempted to say as black as coal!

GIRL MARY

Wreck No :	117	Date Sunk :	10 10 1940
Latitude :	56 01 40 N	Longitude :	03 18 40 W
Decca Lat :	5601.67 N	Decca Long :	0318.67 W
Location :	255°, 4 cables Inchcolm Tower	Area :	Inchcolm
Type :	Drifter	Tonnage :	25 net
Length :	feet Beam : feet	Draught :	feet
How Sunk :	Explosion	Depth :	13 metres

The drifter *Girl Mary* was 25 tons net, probably 70-80 tons gross.

On 10th October 1940 she sank after an explosion, in 7 fathoms (13 metres), 255° 4 cables from Inchcolm Tower, in an area of very poor underwater visibility amongst a tangle of discarded anti-submarine boom netting. Five of the crew were saved, but two were lost. According to Naval records, the explosion was caused by the vessel striking a mine.

THURA

Wreck No :	118	Date Sunk :	13 11 1901
Latitude :	56 00 03 N PA	Longitude :	03 23 00 W PA
Decca Lat :	5600.05 N	Decca Long :	0323.00 W
Location :	Inchgarvie	Area :	Rosyth
Type :	Schooner	Tonnage :	164 gross
Length :	feet Beam : feet	Draught :	feet
How Sunk :	Ran aground	Depth :	metres

On 13th November 1901, the 164 ton Swedish schooner *Thura* was blown on to the rocky island of Inchgarvie, almost under the Forth Bridge, in a severe Easterly gale.

As she was inward bound from Halmstad to Methil with a cargo of pit props, she was obviously driven before the storm for some considerable distance beyond her intended destination before finally striking the rocks.

Inchgarvie is a narrow, elongated rock with a rather pointed Easterly end, and I would expect to find the remains of the *Thura* scattered along the North Eastern edge of the island.

The 1900 edition of *Lloyds Register* lists a *Thuro* and a *Thyra* but no *Thura*.

Thuro was a wooden schooner, 133 tons gross, 83.9 x 21.3 x 10.5 feet built in Denmark in 1877, and registered in Svenborg, Denmark.

Thyra was a 3-masted wooden schooner, 166 tons gross, 96.5 x 21.9 x 11.0 feet, built in 1863 by A.F.H. Conrads of Keil, and registered in Marstal, Denmark

FRI

Wreck No :	119	Date Sunk :	08 1906
Latitude :	56 00 18 N	Longitude :	03 25 00 W
Decca Lat :	5600.30 N	Decca Long :	0325.00 W
Location :	Beamer Rock, near Rosyth	Area :	Rosyth
Type :	Schooner	Tonnage :	495 gross
Length :	138.6 feet Beam : 30.3 feet	Draught :	10.6 feet
How Sunk :	Ran aground	Depth :	metres

The schooner *Fri* of Christiansand was abandoned after running on to Beamer Rock, near the Forth Bridge. The light on the rock was mistaken for the centre light of the bridge.

She was laden with 260 tons of coal, and was on her way to Grangemouth.

Efforts to tow her off resulted in the keel being wrenched away.

The wreck was auctioned at Leith.

Fri was a wooden 3-masted schooner built in 1873 by Hansen of Porsgrund.

HOSIANNA

Wreck No :	120	Date Sunk :	29 10 1889
Latitude :	56 00 18 N	Longitude :	03 24 39 W
Decca Lat :	5600.30 N	Decca Long :	0324.65 W
Location :	Beamer Rock, near Rosyth	Area :	Rosyth
Type :	Schooner	Tonnage :	51 gross
Length :	feet Beam : feet	Draught :	feet
How Sunk :	Ran aground	Depth :	metres

The German wooden schooner *Hosianna* sank after striking *Beimar* rock in 1889 while en route from St. Davids to Varel, Germany with a cargo of coal. The wind at the time was from the South West, Force 2.

That information came from House of Commons Accounts and Papers, 1890-91. How *Hosianna* came to be upriver and upwind of her point of departure, when she should have been going the other way, is not explained!

The spelling of the name of the rock is now *Beamer*, and it is visible at all states of the tide. There is a light at the top of a stone tower built on the rock, which is $^1/_4$ mile upriver from the Forth Road Bridge at 560018N, 032439W.

Depths range from 9 to 27 metres at low water, with overfalls due to the strong tidal streams in the very silty water.

TELESILLA

Wreck No :	121	Date Sunk :	14 09 1896
Latitude :	56 00 22 N	Longitude :	03 24 12 W
Decca Lat :	5600.37 N	Decca Long :	0324.20 W
Location :	Mackintosh Rock, Forth Road Bridge	Area :	Rosyth
Type :	Steamship	Tonnage :	1174 gross
Length :	230.0 feet Beam : 31.6 feet	Draught :	17.3 feet
How Sunk :	Ran aground	Depth :	13 metres

The British iron steamship *Telesilla* was built in 1877 by E. Withy & Co.

Shortly after leaving Grangemouth on 14th September 1896, bound for Hamburg with a cargo of coal, she ran on to Beamer Rock then drifted off to sink adjacent to Mackintosh Rock, which is the rock on which the North towers of the Forth Road Bridge are constructed.

Wreckage was discovered during the construction of the Road Bridge during 1959-1962. On 8th November 1906, it was reported that work involving the removal (or dispersal) of a vessel beached near Queensferry about 9 years previously was going ahead. That report would presumably refer to the *Telesilla*.

SKULDA

Wreck No : 122	Date Sunk : 09 10 1906
Latitude : 56 00 24 N	Longitude : 03 25 05 W
Decca Lat : 5600.40 N	Decca Long : 0325.08 W
Location : Close W of Beamer Rock	Area : Rosyth
Type : Steamship	Tonnage : 1177 gross
Length : 227.0 feet Beam : 33.0 feet	Draught : 14.8 feet
How Sunk : Collision with *Tento*	Depth : 13 metres

This position is very close upriver from Beamer Rock in 13 metres of water.

The British steamship *Skulda*, built in 1882 by S & H Morton of Leith, and belonging to J.T. Salvesen of Grangemouth, sank in collision with the Norwegian steamship *Tento* (541 tons net), in the Firth of Forth while en route from Grangemouth to Stockholm with a general cargo. The collision took place about 100 fathoms (600 feet) West of Beamer Rock.

The *Skulda* was hit practically amidships, near the engine room, and immediately began drifting. It was seen that there was no chance of keeping the vessel afloat, and the *Tento* took off some of the *Skulda*'s 17 crew, while others managed to get away in one of *Skulda*'s boats. The chief officer, who was below at the time of the collision, could not be reached, and went down with the ship. The 16 who were saved were landed at Grangemouth.

The *Tento*, which was built in 1871, was on her way from Norway to Alloa. She sustained considerable damage to her stem, but was able to proceed.

The nature of the damage and the fact that the chief officer could not be rescued before the ship went down suggests that she sank very quickly after the collision, and could not have drifted very far. Three weeks after her sinking, it was reported that her masts and funnel were being removed as they were a danger to shipping.

A large boiler was once awash here at low tide, but is not visible now and may have been scrapped, unless it has merely slipped into deeper water. The size of the boiler suggests this must have been a fairly large steamship.

Strong tidal streams and very silty water make this an unattractive place to investigate at close hand. An additional problem to an on-site search is the MOD police, who patrol this area at the entrance to Rosyth dockyard to prevent unauthorised visitors.

TYR

Wreck No : 123	Date Sunk : 22 07 1900
Latitude : 56 00 27 N PA	Longitude : 03 22 30 W PA
Decca Lat : 5600.45 N	Decca Long : 0322.50 W
Location : ½ mile W of Forth Bridge	Area : Rosyth
Type : Schooner	Tonnage : 158 gross
Length : 88.5 feet Beam : 23.5 feet	Draught : 10.4 feet
How Sunk : Collision with *Achroite*	Depth : metres

While en route from Cockenzie to Grangemouth in ballast, the 158 ton Swedish schooner *Tyr* was lost in collision with the Glasgow steamship *Achroite* $^1/_2$ mile West of the Forth Railway Bridge on 22nd July 1900.

The Tyr was a wooden schooner of 145 tons net, built in 1882 by A.P. Andersen of Figeholm, Sweden.

RUBY

Wreck No :	124	Date Sunk :	10 10 1905
Latitude :	56 00 34 N	Longitude :	03 26 50 W
Decca Lat :	5600.57 N	Decca Long :	0326.83 W
Location :	Off Rosyth	Area :	Rosyth
Type :	Steamship	Tonnage :	481 gross
Length :	175.0 feet Beam : 26.6 feet	Draught :	10.5 feet
How Sunk :	Collision	Depth :	18 metres

The iron steamship *Ruby* is reported to have sunk 2 miles West of the Forth Bridge on 10/10/1905 after colliding with the steamship *Prudhoe Castle* while en route from Middlesbrough to Grangemouth with a cargo of pig iron.

She was reported to lie upside down in 13 fathoms (24 metres), and salvage was abandoned. On 8/11/1906, it was reported that the wreck of the *Ruby* was being removed as she was a danger to shipping. That report must be somewhat inaccurate, as salvage had already been abandoned, and as she lies upside down, her masts and funnel can hardly have been a danger!

The wreck is charted as 17.9 metres in 22 metres. The iron screw steamship *Ruby* was built in 1888 by Scotts of Bowling, and registered in Glasgow.

ELCHO CASTLE

Wreck No :	125	Date Sunk :	Pre-03 1921
Latitude :	56 01 00 N	Longitude :	03 24 48 W
Decca Lat :	5601.00 N	Decca Long :	0324.80 W
Location :	Ashore close to Rosyth Docks	Area :	Rosyth
Type :	Steamship	Tonnage :	
Length :	feet Beam : feet	Draught :	feet
How Sunk :	Foundered	Depth :	metres

The steam collier *Elcho Castle*, laden with coal, foundered in the fairway to Rosyth dockyard shortly after the first world war. She was raised and moved out of the way to a position 1000 feet 300° from Cultness. That would place her in the mud close to the shore at 560100N, 032448W, adjacent to the entrance to the dockyard, and she would presumably have been scrapped at that site, unless it was possible to patch her up and refloat her.

TRIUMPH VI ?

Wreck No : 126	Date Sunk : 15 12 1944
Latitude : 56 02 00 N	Longitude : 03 34 03 W
Decca Lat : 5602.00 N	Decca Long : 0334.07 W
Location : 1¼ miles SW of Crombie Point	Area : Rosyth
Type :	Tonnage : 46 gross
Length : feet Beam : feet	Draught : feet
How Sunk : Collision	Depth : 6 metres

Triumph VI is reported to have been sunk in a collision in the Rosyth area on 15th December 1944.

The position of this wreck, just South of the main channel to Grangemouth, fits the description of the location of its loss 1.25 miles SW of Crombie Point, and suggests that it was most likely the result of a collision, hence I have assumed this to be the *Triumph VI*.

On the other hand, three of the crew of the patrol launch *Mesme* were lost when she was sunk in collision with the submarine *Sunfish* off Grangemouth at 21.30 hrs on 1st September 1940.

Another possibility is that this could be the steam lighter *Glen*, which is thought to have hit a mine between Grangemouth and Crombie on the night of 22nd November 1940. The *Glen* was carrying 5.25" ammunition to Rosyth.

Yet a further possibility is that this might be the 105 ton Norwegian schooner *Sophie*, which was sunk in collision with the Glasgow steamship *Perth* about 2 miles E by N of Bridgeness Pier on 14th October 1898.

CHAPTER 5

THE WRECKS OF KIRKCALDY, METHIL & ELIE

INTRODUCTION

The coastline of this chapter is made up of a mixture of small industrial towns and villages together with more natural scenery. Much of this scenery is relatively low-lying and backed by hills lying inland. Most of the industry is now in decline (such as linoleum manufacture in Kirkcaldy) or has now virtually gone (for example, many coal mines scattered along the coast).

Kirkcaldy is the major town in this area, its water front extending for some five miles. It is one of the largest of a series of small ports on the North side of the Forth. John Paul Jones, the Scottish-born founder of the US Navy, anchored off Kikcaldy in 1779 during the American War of Independence and threatened to attack unless he was given £200,000; this was avoided by the local priest successfully praying on the beach for a violent offshore wind to drive the raiders out to sea!

Methil lies seven miles to the East of Kirkcaldy along a coast riddled with caves. It was an important convoy marshalling centre during both World Wars; nowadays it is a centre for the oil-rig building industry.

Lower Largo lies between Methil and Elie and its claim to fame is that it was the birthplace of Alexander Selkirk, the real Robinson Crusoe, and his statue can be seen near the seafront. It is well worth walking up the 952 feet high hill of Largo Law behind the village as this offers superb views of the Fife coast and the Firth of Forth.

Elie is now quite a popular resort having been developed around the original 16th-century fishing harbour.

It may be possible to launch relatively small inflatables at Elie, but there are no other launching sites along this stretch of the north shore of the Forth. The nearest places to launch are Kinghorn and Burntisland to the west, and Anstruther to the east.

Kirkcaldy, Methil and Elie area

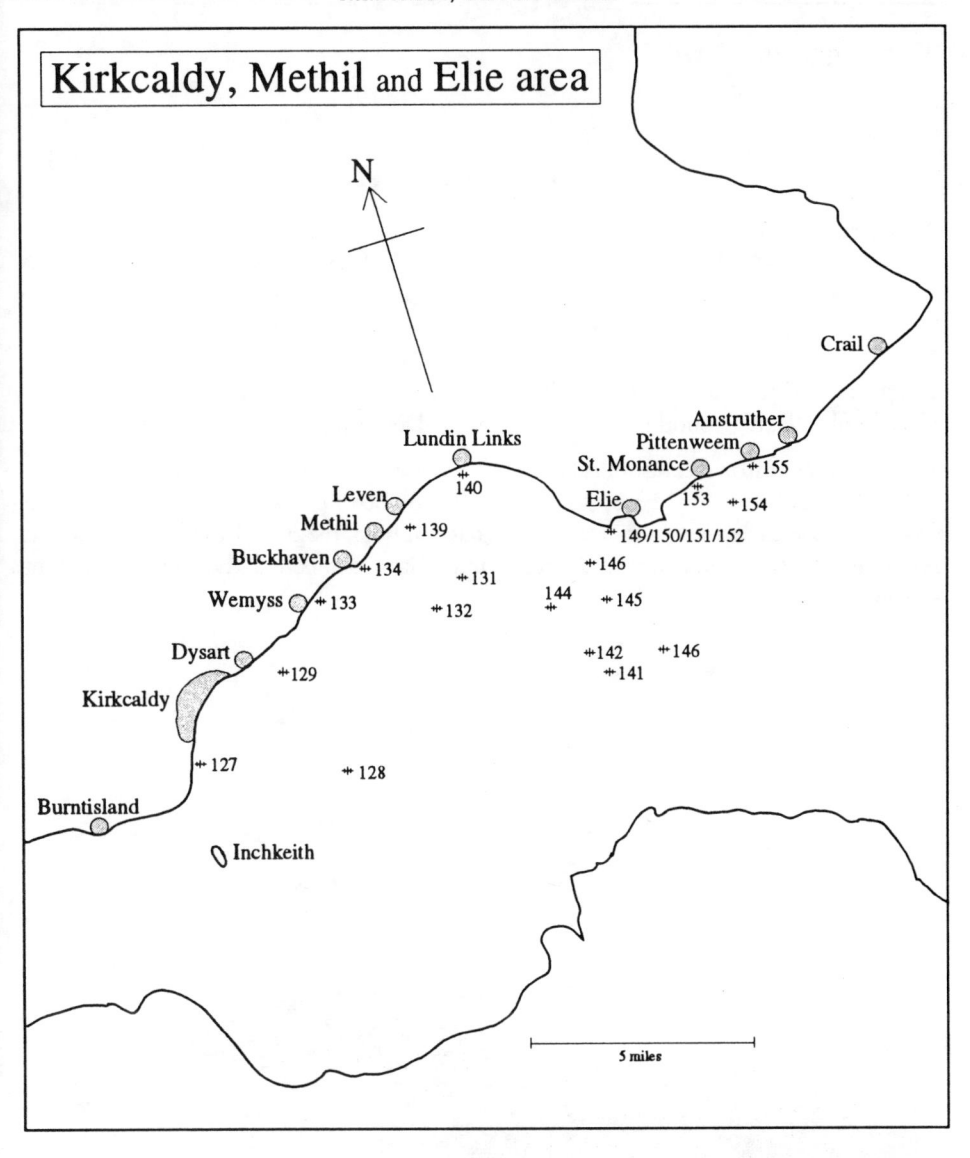

Chart showing the location of wrecks lying off the South coast of Fife between Kirkcaldy and Pittenweem.

The Wrecks

ADAM SMITH

Wreck No : 127
Latitude : 56 05 36 N PA
Decca Lat : 5605.60 N
Location : Long Craig Rock, Kirkcaldy
Type : Steamship
Length : 150.3 feet Beam : 22.1 feet
How Sunk : Ran aground

Date Sunk : 26 12 1884
Longitude : 03 09 00 W PA
Decca Long : 0309.00 W
Area : Kirkcaldy
Tonnage : 185 gross
Draught : 12.0 feet
Depth : metres

The 159 ton net iron steamship *Adam Smith* was built at Port Glasgow in 1876.

When returning to her home port from London on Boxing Day 1884, she ran on to Long Craig Rock, a little over a mile South of Kirkcaldy Harbour and became a total loss. Although no lives were lost, this event must have dampened the crew's Christmas somewhat!

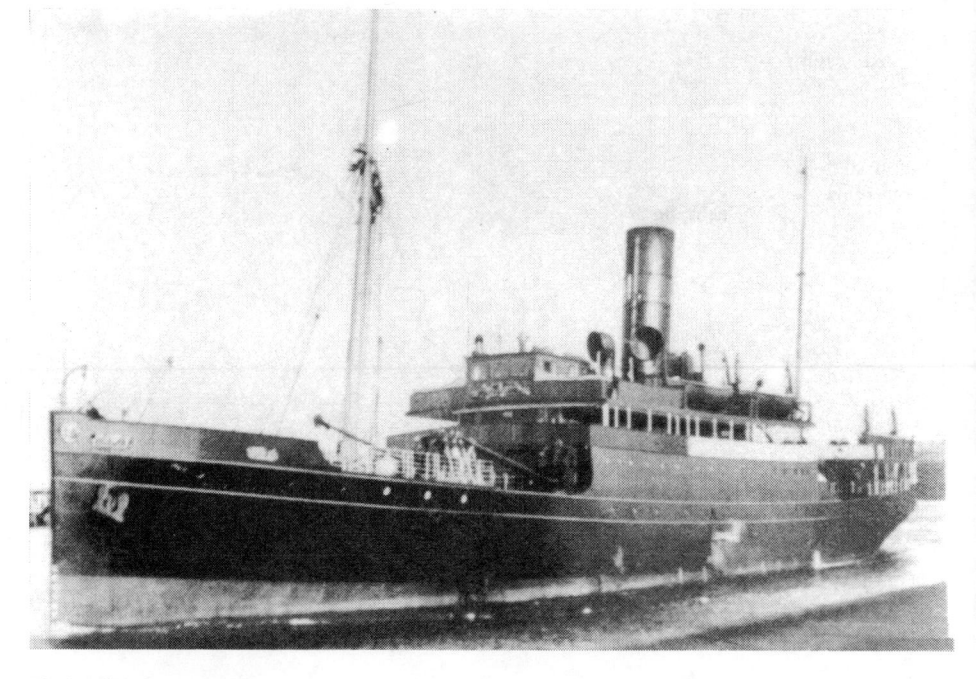

The Royal Archer
(photograph courtesy of the
executors of P. Ransome-Wallis).

ROYAL ARCHER

Wreck No :	128	Date Sunk :	24 02 1940
Latitude :	56 06 26 N	Longitude :	02 59 56 W
Decca Lat :	5606.43 N	Decca Long :	0259.93 W
Location :	5 miles ESE of Kirkcaldy	Area :	Kirkcaldy
Type :	Steamship	Tonnage :	2266 gross
Length :	290.5 feet Beam : 41.2 feet	Draught :	18.0 feet
How Sunk :	Mined	Depth :	24 metres

Built in 1928 by Scotts of Greenock, the *Royal Archer* was mined while en route from London to Leith with 630 tons of general cargo. All 27 crew and one gunner were saved.

Her position was reported as 6 miles 44.5° from Inchkeith Lighthouse, and charted at 560618N, 025956W (14.4 metres in 24 metres).

She was dived on just West of the charted position in 1982, and was found to be in a somewhat broken up state. Parts seen stood 3 to 4 metres high in general depths of 27 metres.

In 1984 Decca co-ordinates were given as Red G 16.6, Green E 46.95. This plots in 560622N, 030005W.- i.e. 5606.37N, 0300.08W.

UNKNOWN - PRE 1946

Wreck No :	129	Date Sunk :	Pre - 1946
Latitude :	56 07 23 N	Longitude :	03 05 23 W
Decca Lat :	5607.38 N	Decca Long :	0305.38 W
Location :	2 miles E of Kirkcaldy	Area :	Kirkcaldy
Type :	Barge	Tonnage :	
Length :	feet Beam : feet	Draught :	feet
How Sunk :		Depth :	9 metres

In 1946 and again in 1947, the wreck of a barge was reported 1 mile E of Dysart and 2 miles from Kirkcaldy pier at 560727N, 030518W. This was subsequently amended in 1959 to 560723N, 030523W.

The wreck stands only about 2 feet up from the bottom in about 10 metres depth.

UNKNOWN

Wreck No :	130	Date Sunk :	
Latitude :	56 08 18 N	Longitude :	02 58 21 W
Decca Lat :	5608.30 N	Decca Long :	0258.35 W
Location :	2.75 miles SSE of Methil	Area :	Methil
Type :	Steamship	Tonnage :	
Length :	feet Beam : feet	Draught :	feet

How Sunk :		Depth :	25 metres

This is obviously the remains of an old steamship, as wreckage including a boiler standing up 3 metres high in a general depth of 32 metres was found when dived in 1988.

The position was given as Decca Red G 15.13, Green F 33.01, which converts to 560818N, 025821W, where it is charted as a wreck at 27 metres in 32 metres.

UNKNOWN

Wreck No :	131	Date Sunk :	1970-1971
Latitude :	56 08 58 N	Longitude :	02 56 57 W
Decca Lat :	5608.97 N	Decca Long :	0256.95 W
Location :	2.75 miles SE of Methil	Area :	Methil
Type :	Barge	Tonnage :	
Length :	30.0 feet Beam : feet	Draught :	feet
How Sunk :		Depth :	24 metres

A wooden barge about 30 feet long, standing 2 metres high, laden with steel scaffolding, was reported to have sunk while engaged in repair work on a moored oil rig in 1970 or 1971.

CHARLES HAMMOND ?

Wreck No :	132	Date Sunk :	02 11 1918
Latitude :	56 09 05 N	Longitude :	02 57 31 W
Decca Lat :	5609.08 N	Decca Long :	0257.52 W
Location :	2.5 miles SE of Methil	Area :	Methil
Type :	Trawler	Tonnage :	324 gross
Length :	feet Beam : feet	Draught :	feet
How Sunk :	Collision with *Marksman*	Depth :	22 metres

When dived on in 1988, the wreck charted in 26 metres at 560905N, 025731W was found to be an old steamship or steam trawler, with the highest point standing 4 metres up from the bottom. Could this be the steam trawler *Charles Hammond* which was sunk off Kirkcaldy in a collision with HMS *Marksman* on 2nd November 1918?

A W SINGLETON

Wreck No :	133	Date Sunk :	18 10 1898
Latitude :	56 09 30 N PA	Longitude :	03 03 30 W PA
Decca Lat :	5609.50 N	Decca Long :	0303.50 W
Location :	On rocks near Wemyss Castle	Area :	Methil
Type :	Barque	Tonnage :	546 gross

Length :	feet	Beam :	feet	Draught : feet
How Sunk :	Ran aground			Depth : 3 metres

The Norwegian barque *A W Singleton*, en route from Gothenburg to Methil with a cargo of pit props, was blown on to rocks near Wemyss Castle by an Easterly storm on 18th October 1898, and was totally wrecked.

There is unlikely to be much left intact, but access is easy, and it may be worth a look to see what remains to be picked up.

THORGNY

Wreck No :	134	Date Sunk :	03 11 1899
Latitude :	56 10 12 N PA	Longitude :	03 01 30 W PA
Decca Lat :	5610.20 N	Decca Long :	0301.50 W
Location :	Near Buckhaven	Area :	Methil
Type :	Barque	Tonnage :	461 gross
Length :	137.1 feet Beam : 30.1 feet	Draught :	16.6 feet
How Sunk :	Ran aground	Depth :	metres

The 461 ton Norwegian wooden barque *Thorgny*, built in 1876, was driven on to the rocks near Buckhaven by a severe SSW gale on 3rd November 1899.

ANTELOPE

Wreck No :	135	Date Sunk :	22 02 1888
Latitude :	56 10 30 N PA	Longitude :	03 00 45 W PA
Decca Lat :	5610.50 N	Decca Long :	0300.75 W
Location :	Stranded at Methil	Area :	Methil
Type :	Steamship	Tonnage :	509 gross
Length :	feet Beam : feet	Draught :	feet
How Sunk :	Ran aground	Depth :	metres

The West Hartlepool iron steamship *Antelope*, en route from Methil to Aalborg, ran aground on leaving Methil harbour on 22nd February 1888, and became a total loss.

SCIO

Wreck No :	136	Date Sunk :	27 11 1881
Latitude :	56 10 30 N PA	Longitude :	03 01 00 W PA
Decca Lat :	5610.50 N	Decca Long :	0301.00 W
Location :	near Methil	Area :	Methil
Type :	Brig	Tonnage :	266 gross

Length :	94.4 feet	Beam : 27.0 feet	Draught :	16.2	feet
			Depth :		metres
How Sunk :	Ran aground				

The 266 ton brig *Scio*, left South Shields for Copenhagen, but was blown off course by a South West gale, and became a total loss when she ran ashore near Methil on 27th November 1881.

NO. 4 HOPPER

Wreck No :	137	Date Sunk :	07 12 1908
Latitude :	56 10 50 N PA	Longitude :	03 00 30 W PA
Decca Lat :	5610.83 N	Decca Long :	0300.50 W
Location :	On rocks near Methil breakwater	Area :	Methil
Type :	Dredger	Tonnage :	265 gross
Length :	feet Beam : feet	Draught :	feet
How Sunk :	Ran aground	Depth :	1 metres

Steam dredger *No. 4* went ashore on rocks near Methil breakwater where she later broke up and became a total loss. She was 179 tons net.

ASHGROVE

Wreck No :	138	Date Sunk :	16 01 1912
Latitude :	56 11 00 N	Longitude :	03 00 12 W
Decca Lat :	5611.00 N	Decca Long :	0300.20 W
Location :	On Sea Wall at Methil	Area :	Methil
Type :	Steamship	Tonnage :	1702 gross
Length :	285.3 feet Beam : 34.6 feet	Draught :	17.7 feet
How Sunk :	Ran aground	Depth :	1 metres

The 1079 tons net iron screw steamer *Ashgrove* built in 1882 by Earle's Co., Hull, was driven on to the sea wall at Methil and became a total loss. Three of her crew were lost.

The ship had been en route from Middlesbrough to Methil in ballast.

KAREN

Wreck No :	139	Date Sunk :	05 02 1940
Latitude :	56 11 04 N	Longitude :	02 58 45 W
Decca Lat :	5611.07 N	Decca Long :	0258.75 W
Location :	1 mile E of Methil	Area :	Methil
Type :	Auxiliary motor schooner	Tonnage :	331 gross
Length :	130.0 feet Beam : 29.0 feet	Draught :	13.0 feet
How Sunk :		Depth :	5 metres

RAP

Wreck No :	140	Date Sunk :	05 11 1911
Latitude :	56 12 30 N PA	Longitude :	02 57 00 W PA
Decca Lat :	5612.50 N	Decca Long :	0257.00 W
Location :	Stranded at Lundin Links	Area :	Methil
Type :	Schooner	Tonnage :	132 gross
Length :	93.3 feet Beam : 23.8 feet	Draught :	10.7 feet
How Sunk :	Ran aground	Depth :	metres

The Norwegian schooner *Rap* of 116 tons net, was reported to have stranded at Lundin Links, Largo Bay on 5th November 1911. She was built at Bergen in 1882.

Another schooner named *Rap* was reported to have been lost by stranding at Randerston on 20th March 1879.

MARE VIVIMUS

Wreck No :	141	Date Sunk :	12 12 1925
Latitude :	56 08 00 N	Longitude :	02 51 00 W
Decca Lat :	5608.00 N	Decca Long :	0251.00 W
Location :	3.25 miles S of Kincraig Point	Area :	Elie
Type :	Trawler	Tonnage :	82 gross
Length :	78.0 feet Beam : 19.0 feet	Draught :	9.0 feet
How Sunk :	Foundered	Depth :	44 metres

Mare Vivimus was a steam trawler sunk in 1925.

Although charted in 560800N, 025100W, this is obviously an approximate position, and it was not found during an asdic search in 1960.

ROLFSBORG

Wreck No :	142	Date Sunk :	13 07 1945
Latitude :	56 08 13 N	Longitude :	02 52 03 W
Decca Lat :	5608.22 N	Decca Long :	0252.05 W
Location :	3.25 miles SW of Elie	Area :	Elie
Type :	Steamship	Tonnage :	1831 gross
Length :	264.4 feet Beam : 42.0 feet	Draught :	18.0 feet
How Sunk :	Collision with *Empire Swordsman*	Depth :	27 metres

The *Rolfsborg* was a steel collier built in 1915 at Fredrikstad, Finland. She sank following a collision with SS *Empire Swordsman*. In 1945 she was located at 560816N, 025215W.

In 1960 she was located at 560817N, 025155W. In 1987 she was located at 560813N, 025203W. Another position nearby at 560814N, 025220W may also be worth checking.

She is apparently intact, lying on her port side, and standing 12 metres high in 40 metres. A very large brass eagle is fastened around the stern.

UNKNOWN - PRE 1940

Wreck No :	143	Date Sunk :	Pre-1940
Latitude :	56 08 22 N	Longitude :	02 48 51 W
Decca Lat :	5608.37 N	Decca Long :	0248.85 W
Location :	2.75 miles S of Chapel Ness	Area :	Elie
Type :		Tonnage :	
Length :	feet Beam : feet	Draught :	feet
How Sunk :		Depth :	50 metres

A fisherman's fastener known locally as *Rocky Mill* was reported in 1977 in Decca chain 3, Green C38.5, Purple 1C66.7, which converts to 560816N, 024851W.

In 1984 an obstruction was located but not investigated at 560822N, 024851W. *Rocky Mill* has also been reported in Decca chain 3, Green C37.2, Purple 1C68.8.

Two obstructions were reported in position 560833N, 024924W in 1939, but apparently a decision was taken in 1940 to record them as one wreck at 560830N, 024930W PA, which is a convenient, tidy round number, but no wreck is marked on the chart in or near that position, and in 1959, the survey vessel *HMS Scott* was unable to find any wreck there.

Is the obstruction located in 1984, and *Rocky Mill* one wreck broken in two pieces, or are there really two wrecks?

UNKNOWN - PRE 1939

Wreck No :	144	Date Sunk :	Pre-1939
Latitude :	56 09 17 N	Longitude :	02 52 51 W
Decca Lat :	5609.28 N	Decca Long :	0252.87 W
Location :	2 miles SSW of Kincraig Point	Area :	Elie
Type :		Tonnage :	
Length :	feet Beam : feet	Draught :	feet
How Sunk :		Depth :	32 metres

In 1939, a non-sub contact was reported at 560912N, 025340W, two miles SSW of Kincraig Point. It was not located in that position in 1959 by *HMS Scott*, but a wreck was found at 560919N, 025340W, with a least depth of 27 metres, standing up 6 metres in a depth of 33 metres. As a result, it was charted as a wreck at 27 metres in that position.

Almost 30 years later, it could not be found there, despite repeated searches around the area in 1987 and 1988, but wreckage standing 3 metres high in a general depth of 38 metres was located half a mile to the East at 560917N, 025251W.

These are all probably the same wreck, the differing positions stemming from the development over the years of more accurate position fixing equipment. (See wreck in position 560822N, 024851W).

PHAEACIAN

Wreck No :	145	Date Sunk :	29 09 1943
Latitude :	56 09 20 N	Longitude :	02 5**]** 32 W
Decca Lat :	5609.33 N	Decca Long :	0251.53 W
Location :	2 miles S of Kincraig Point	Area :	Elie
Type :	Steamship	Tonnage :	480 gross
Length :	144.1 feet Beam : 25.2 feet	Draught :	11.1 feet
How Sunk :	Collision with *San Zotico*	Depth :	22 metres

The Harwich-registered steel screw, three-masted steamship *Phaeacian* was built in 1920 by Mistley S.B. & Rprg. Co.

On 29th March 1943 she was in collision with the British steam tanker *San Zotico*, and sank shortly after being taken in tow by a tug.

In 1986 she was reported to be broken into three parts which stand no more than 4 metres high in general depths of 30 metres.

The position was originally recorded as 560924N, 025142W, but she is now charted at 560920N, 025132W, two miles South of Kincraig Point near Elie.

UNKNOWN - PRE 1940

Wreck No :	146	Date Sunk :	
Latitude :	56 09 39 N	Longitude :	02 53 19 W
Decca Lat :	5609.65 N	Decca Long :	0253.32 W
Location :	1.75 miles SSW Kincraig Point	Area :	Elie
Type :		Tonnage :	
Length : feet Beam : feet		Draught : feet	
How Sunk :		Depth :	24 metres

This may be part of the wreck at 560943N, 025314W, (5609.72N, 0253.23W), or the wreck charted at 560942N, 025318W. (5609.70N, 0253.30W).

In 1960 small obstructions close together were reported to stand up 2 metres from the bottom in a depth of 25 metres.

UNKNOWN - U-BOAT ?

Wreck No :	147	Date Sunk :	Pre-1922
Latitude :	56 09 45 N	Longitude :	02 50 45 W
Decca Lat :	5609.75 N	Decca Long :	0250.75 W

Location :	1.5 miles SSW of Kincraig Point	**Area :**		Elie
Type :	Submarine ?	**Tonnage :**		
Length :	feet **Beam :** feet	**Draught :**		feet
How Sunk :		**Depth :**		25 metres

The master of the steamer *Britannic* reported passing a *shoal sunken wreck* (whatever that might be), or submerged object at 560945N, 025045W on 25/10/1922.

I would have been inclined to disregard this one because:
1) of the date - position fixing at that time was considerably less accurate than today, 70 years on, although as this location is not very far from shore, reasonably accurate bearings of points on the land might have been taken, and
2) this was long before the days of echo sounders - what was used to detect a wreck in those days?

I do, however, have three reasons for including this position:
1) The Navy's Hydrographic Department placed sufficient credence in the report to include it in the obstruction register, although it is not charted.
2) When I plotted it on my chart, it turned out to be very close to the position another informant had marked as a possible sunken U-Boat!
3) Yet another informant has suggested the possibility that this may be a Dutch submarine from which bodies were recovered before the wreck was dispersed with explosives - (see *O-13*) - although the *O-13* was sunk in 1940.

ARIZONA

Wreck No :	148	**Date Sunk :**	29 09 1940
Latitude :	56 10 14 N	**Longitude :**	02 52 23 W
Decca Lat :	5610.23 N	**Decca Long :**	0252.38 W
Location :	1 mile SSW of Kincraig Point	**Area :**	Elie
Type :	Motor vessel	**Tonnage :**	398 gross
Length :	143.4 feet **Beam :** 26.2 feet	**Draught :**	8.9 feet
How Sunk :	Mined	**Depth :**	12 metres

The Dutch motor vessel *Arizona*, built in 1939, was mined while en route from Methil with a cargo of 500 tons of coal. Five of the crew of eight were lost.

In 1984 the wreck was reported to be well dispersed with the highest points standing 4 to 5 metres up from the bottom, 204° 1 mile from Kincraig Point signal tower, or 2 miles South of Elie Ness.

VULCAN

Wreck No :	149	**Date Sunk :**	15 10 1882
Latitude :	56 10 45 N PA	**Longitude :**	02 50 30 W PA
Decca Lat :	5610.75 N	**Decca Long :**	0250.50 W
Location :	Vows Rocks, Elie	**Area :**	Elie

Type :	Steamship	Tonnage :	235 gross
Length :	141.0 feet Beam : 22.2 feet	Draught :	12.5 feet
How Sunk :	Ran aground	Depth :	5 metres

In a Force 10 Southerly storm on 15th October 1882 the iron steamship *Vulcan* was blown on to Vows Rocks off Elie, while en route from Middlesbrough to Grangemouth with a cargo of pig iron and two passengers. Five lives were lost, along with the ship.

The report does not specify whether the vessel hit the East or the West Vows, which are about half a mile apart. The vessel was built in 1874 by R. Dixon of Middlesbrough.

GRAF TOTLEBEN

Wreck No :	150	Date Sunk :	20 02 1912
Latitude :	56 10 50 N	Longitude :	02 50 00 W
Decca Lat :	5610.83 N	Decca Long :	0250.00 W
Location :	At East Vows, Elie	Area :	Elie
Type :	Steamship	Tonnage :	1484 gross
Length :	246.0 feet Beam : 33.3 feet	Draught :	17.6 feet
How Sunk :	Ran aground	Depth :	3 metres

Graf Totleben was a Russian iron steamship of 791 tons net en route from Methil to Riga with a cargo of coal and one passenger. She had a crew of 17. No lives were lost, but the vessel was stranded and became a total loss.

Graf Totleben (ex-*Skjold*) was built in 1881 by Lobnitz of Renfrew.

JUPITER

Wreck No :	151	Date Sunk :	24 09 1897
Latitude :	56 11 00 N PA	Longitude :	02 48 30 W PA
Decca Lat :	5611.00 N	Decca Long :	0258.50 W
Location :	Elie Ness	Area :	Elie
Type :	Schooner	Tonnage :	326 gross
Length :	feet Beam : feet	Draught :	feet
How Sunk :	Ran aground	Depth :	metres

The 326 ton Russian schooner *Jupiter* was lost on the rocks at Elieness on 24th September 1897, en route from Alloa to Riga, Latvia. with a cargo of coal. She ran ashore on the rocks to the East of Fish Rock, and the local lifesaving brigade were soon on the scene with their rocket apparatus. Five of the crew of seven were taken off by breeches buoy, but the captain, who was the owner of the vessel, and the mate, refused to leave. They stated that they would prefer to go down with the ship, which lay in several fathoms of water, grinding heavily on the rocks.

Consideration was given to removing them forcibly from the vessel, but this was not resorted to, and it is not known whether the captain and mate subsequently changed their minds, or if they did go down with the ship.

THE BRODERS

Wreck No : 152			**Date Sunk :** 07 10 1897	
Latitude : 56 11 00 N PA			**Longitude :** 02 48 30 W PA	
Decca Lat : 5611.00 N			**Decca Long :** 0248.50 W	
Location : Elie Ness			**Area :** Elie	
Type : Lighter			**Tonnage :** 160 gross	
Length : feet	**Beam :**	feet	**Draught :**	feet
How Sunk : Ran aground			**Depth :**	metres

The Grangemouth lighter *The Broders* was engaged in salvage work, and was moored over the wreck of the *Jupiter* at Elieness.

During a WSW Force 7 near gale on 7th October 1897, she was blown ashore at the same place as the *Jupiter*, and joined her on the bottom.

ANSGAR

Wreck No : 153			**Date Sunk :** 13 02 1910	
Latitude : 56 11 42 N			**Longitude :** 02 47 00 W	
Decca Lat : 5611.70 N			**Decca Long :** 0247.00 W	
Location : Near Ardross Castle, near St. Monance			**Area :** Elie	
Type : Steamship			**Tonnage :** 1347 gross	
Length : 235.8 feet	**Beam :** 33.1 feet		**Draught :** 15.8 feet	
How Sunk : Ran aground			**Depth :** 6 metres	

Ansgar was a Danish iron steamship built in 1879 by Burmeister & Wain of Copenhagen.

DANTE

Wreck No : 154	**Date Sunk :** 25 10 1883
Latitude : 56 12 00 N PA	**Longitude :** 02 46 00 W PA
Decca Lat : 5612.00 N	**Decca Long :** 0246.00 W
Location : 7 miles W by S of Fife Ness	**Area :** Elie
Type : Brigantine	**Tonnage :** 177 gross

Length :	107.1 feet	Beam : 21.7 feet	Draught :	13.1	feet
How Sunk :	Foundered		Depth :		metres

The wooden brigantine *Dante* is reported to have foundered in a storm 7 miles West by South of Fife Ness on 25th October 1883. She had been en route from Teignmouth to Leith with a cargo of China clay.

There must be an error in that position description, (which was given in *Parliamentary Papers*), because it plots about a mile inland from St. Monance!

I have not checked the newspapers of the following days for a report, but anyone who cares to do so might be rewarded with information which could lead to finding this wreck! The approximate lat./long. position given above is off St. Monance, but has been given only as a convenient *parking place* until further information is forthcoming to establish a more accurate position.

GARELOCH

Wreck No :	155	Date Sunk :	18 08 1935
Latitude :	56 12 30 N	Longitude :	02 44 00 W
Decca Lat :	5612.50 N	Decca Long :	0244.00 W
Location :	Billowness, Pittenweem	Area :	Elie
Type :	Trawler	Tonnage :	246 gross
Length :	feet Beam : feet	Draught :	feet
How Sunk :	Ran aground	Depth :	4 metres

The 246 ton Aberdeen steam trawler *Gareloch* (ex-*Lily Melling* of Fleetwood), ran aground near Anstruther bathing pool in dense fog on the morning of 18th August, 1935.

She had loaded over 100 tons of coal at Methil and was on her way back to Aberdeen with a skeleton crew when she ran aground and was badly holed. When the tide receded she heeled sharply over on her port side, and one member of the crew was thrown on to the rocks, sustaining two broken ribs.

The trawler lay so close to the shore that a number of visitors to the swimming pool swam out and boarded the vessel. With the return of the high tide in the evening she could not be refloated.

A photograph in the *Dundee Courier* of 19th August 1935 shows the trawler lying on her port side on the rocks at Billowness, Anstruther. The tide has receded leaving only the bottom of the keel and her rudder touching the water. The rest of the vessel is high and dry.

Chapter 6

The Wrecks of the Isle of May

Introduction

The May is the biggest island in the Forth, and is a major bird sanctuary. It is a mile long rock with 150 feet high cliffs along its western side, while its eastern side is low-lying. There are several caves along its coastline together with off-lying reefs.

The first lighthouse in Scotland was constructed on the island in 1636. It was known as *The Beacon*, and its coal fire in a large iron basket on the flat roof, consumed from 1 ton of coal per night in the summer, to 3 tons per night during the longer winter nights. The remains of this old lighthouse are still visible.

During the construction of the lighthouse, the architect was drowned in one of the sudden, unpredictable storms for which the Forth is notorious, and Eppie Laing, an Anstruther woman, was burned at the stake, having been accused of causing the storm by witchcraft!

The cost of operating that light was offset by taxes on vessels using the Forth ports. Foreign ships paid a tax twice the amount imposed on Scottish ships. Despite the Union of the Crowns in 1603, English ships were classed as foreign!

The present lighthouse, *The Tower*, was built in 1816. It shines out from 240 feet above sea level and is visible for some 26 miles, emphasising the danger of the May to shipping.

The Isle of May offers some of the best diving in the Forth and, consequently, is much visited by many diving clubs. Underwater visibility is generally considerably better than at many other locations in the Forth. Additionally, very many vessels have been lost both along its shoreline and in its vicinity. Wreckage from both wartime and peacetime shipping casualties is strewn around the island, especially among the shallows of the East coast, and some of the wreckage is visible on the shore.

Anstruther, 5 miles to the North West, is the nearest effective launching site for the Isle of May. Like all other harbours in the area, Anstruther is tidal and is thus best used at mid-tide (allowing time for a dive, followed by a recovery at the next mid-tide).

The Isle of May

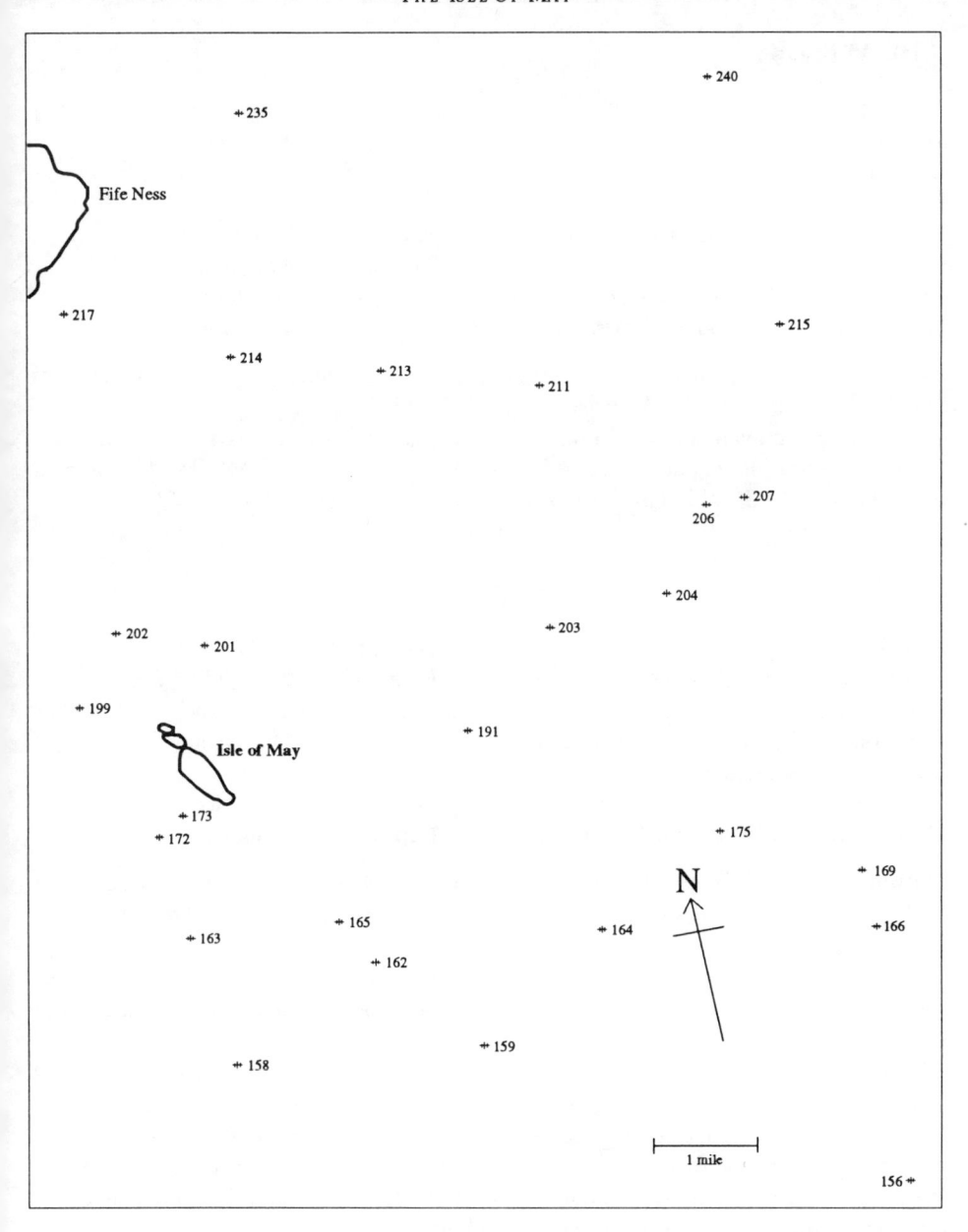

Chart showing the locations of the wrecks lying in the vicinity of the Isle of May. The area covered extends from some five miles East north east of Fife Ness to some eight miles North of North Berwick

The Wrecks

U-12

Wreck No:	156	Date Sunk:	10 03 1915
Latitude:	56 07 12 N	Longitude:	02 20 00 W
Decca Lat:	5607.20 N	Decca Long:	0220.00 W
Location:	8 miles SE of May Island	Area:	May Island
Type:	Submarine	Tonnage:	493 gross
Length:	188.3 feet Beam: 18.7 feet	Draught:	10.2 feet
How Sunk:	Rammed by HMS Ariel	Depth:	55 metres

This class of U-boat displaced 493 tons surfaced, 611 tons submerged. *U-12* (Kratzsch) was rammed by the destroyer HMS *Ariel*.

Curiously, Dan van der Vat, in his book *The Atlantic Campaign*, says *U-12*, under the newly promoted commander Weddigen, was rammed and sunk by HMS *Dreadnought* near Scapa Flow on 18/3/1915. This is incorrect. It was actually the *U-29*.

ALEKTO

Wreck No:	157	Date Sunk:	18 09 1898
Latitude:	56 07 35 N PA	Longitude:	02 39 50 W PA
Decca Lat:	5607.58 N	Decca Long:	0239.83 W
Location:	5 miles WSW of May Island	Area:	May Island
Type:	Schooner	Tonnage:	91 gross
Length:	feet Beam: feet	Draught:	feet
How Sunk:	Collision with *Ben Macdui*	Depth:	40 metres

Outward bound from Bo'ness to Christiansand with a cargo of coal the Norwegian schooner *Alekto* was run down by a steamship between the Bass Rock and May Island in the early hours of 18th September 1898.

Although the steamer's lights had been plainly seen, the collision was of such a force that the schooner's bows were almost entirely smashed, and the foremast fell across the lifeboat on the deck.

The steamer kept on its course after the collision and Captain Anderson and his crew were taken off by another Norwegian schooner, which was also bound from the Forth to Christiansand with coal. Captain Anderson deemed it advisable to go to Leith to report the matter and try to identify the colliding steamer. With two members of his crew he transferred to the inward-bound Granton steam trawler *St. Bernard*, the remainder of his crew remaining aboard their homeward-bound rescuer's vessel.

Shortly after the crew boarded the *St. Bernard*, the Alekto foundered about 5 miles WSW of the May Island.

The colliding vessel was subsequently identified as the Belgian steamship *Ben Macdui*.

UNKNOWN - Pre 1919

Wreck No : 158	Date Sunk : Pre-1919
Latitude : 56 08 18 N	Longitude : 02 32 40 W
Decca Lat : 5608.30 N	Decca Long : 0232.67 W
Location : 2.5 miles S of May Island	Area : May Island
Type :	Tonnage :
Length : feet Beam : feet	Draught : feet
How Sunk :	Depth : 45 metres

This is an unknown wreck sunk pre-1919.

UNKNOWN

Wreck No : 159	Date Sunk :
Latitude : 56 08 30 N PA	Longitude : 02 28 18 W PA
Decca Lat : 5608.50 N	Decca Long : 0228.30 W
Location : 3.5 miles SE of May Island	Area : May Island
Type :	Tonnage :
Length : feet Beam : feet	Draught : feet
How Sunk :	Depth : 49 metres

Charted as Wk PA with at least 35 metres clearance in a general depth of 49 metres.

UNKNOWN - UB-63?

Wreck No : 160	Date Sunk :
Latitude : 56 08 57 N	Longitude : 01 54 30 W
Decca Lat : 5608.95 N	Decca Long : 0154.50 W
Location : 16 miles 38° St. Abbs Head	Area : May Island
Type :	Tonnage :
Length : feet Beam : feet	Draught : feet
How Sunk :	Depth : 48 metres

Charted as a wreck, this position is only 3.5 miles from the approximate position given for the sinking of UB-63, depth charged by HM Trawlers on 28/1/1918.

UNKNOWN - WW2

Wreck No : 161	Date Sunk : WW2
Latitude : 56 09 00 N PA	Longitude : 02 38 00 W PA

SHIPWRECKS OF THE FORTH

Decca Lat :	5609.00 N		Decca Long :	0238.00 W
Location :	3.25 miles WSW of May Island		Area :	May Island
Type :			Tonnage :	
Length :	feet Beam :		feet Draught :	feet
How Sunk :			Depth :	47 metres

An unknown WW2 loss is thought to lie in this approximate position.

AVONDALE PARK

Wreck No :	162	Date Sunk :	07 05 1945
Latitude :	56 09 17 N	Longitude :	02 30 08 W
Decca Lat :	5609.28 N	Decca Long :	0230.13 W
Location :	1.5 miles SE of May Island	Area :	May Island
Type :	Steamship	Tonnage :	2878 gross
Length :	320.1 feet Beam : 49.5 feet	Draught :	23.1 feet
How Sunk :	Torpedoed by *U-2336*	Depth :	45 metres

According to *Lloyds* the *Avondale Park* was sunk 1 mile SE of May Island while en route from Hull to Belfast.

The wreck charted at 560917N, 023008W was first located by *HMS Scott* in 1962, and was reported in 1965 to have a least depth of 44.5 metres, standing some 10 metres above the seabed which is at 55 metres, and gave the impression of being a large wreck, about 350 feet long.

When dived in 1992, she was found to be lying with a list to starboard.

Avondale Park was the last British ship to be sunk in the Second World War. The torpedoing by *U-2336* took place at 23.00 hrs on the last day of the war, after the German surrender documents had been signed, but before the time of their effect at midnight on the 7th, despite an order issued to U-Boats on 4th May not to carry out any more attacks in view of the impending German surrender. Two of the crew of this Canadian-built vessel were lost out of a total of 28 crew and 4 gunners. The Type XXIII U-Boat *U-2336*, returned to its base unscathed and later surrendered to the British. Kapitanleutnant Emil Klusemeir, who had been on his first operational patrol as captain, claimed that he had not received the orders to cease fire broadcast by U-Boat HQ on the 4th.

During the course of my research for this book, I met Andrew Jeffrey, the author of *This Dangerous Menace* - the story of Dundee and the River Tay at War. He was in the course of doing research for his next book, *This Present Emergency*, which covers the same subject in relation to the River Forth, and we met to see if we had uncovered material which may be useful to each other. I told him about Klusemeir sinking the *Avondale Park* and *Sneland I* in the last hour of the war. In a subsequent conversation with the Earl of Elgin, Andrew Jeffrey related this story to His Grace, who was most interested to discover why he had been prevented that night 47 years ago, from lighting the bonfire he had prepared at his Broomhall Estate near Rosyth, to celebrate the end of the war!

COLUMBA

Wreck No :	163	Date Sunk :	10 03 1918
Latitude :	56 09 30 N	Longitude :	02 33 30 W
Decca Lat :	5609.50 N	Decca Long :	0233.50 W
Location :	1.5 miles SSW of S tip of May Island	Area :	May Island
Type :	Trawler	Tonnage :	138 gross
Length : 100.0 feet	Beam : 20.1 feet	Draught :	10.1 feet
How Sunk :	Mined	Depth :	49 metres

The steam trawler *Columba* was a 138 tons gross iron screw ketch built in 1893 by Hawthorns of Leith.

She was requisitioned by the Navy during the first world war, and was sunk by a mine on 10th March 1918. In 1968 the position was given as 560910N, 023248W and charted as PA on chart No. 175 published 1981, but has since been altered to 560930N, 023330W, 1.5 miles SSW of the South tip of May Island.

BEN ATTOW

Wreck No :	164	Date Sunk :	27 02 1940
Latitude :	56 09 36 N	Longitude :	02 26 00 W
Decca Lat :	5609.60 N	Decca Long :	0226.00 W
Location :	4 miles 120° S. Ness May Island	Area :	May Island
Type :	Trawler	Tonnage :	156 gross
Length : 115.5 feet	Beam : 22.1 feet	Draught :	11.9 feet
How Sunk :	Mined	Depth :	48 metres

The *Ben Attow* was a steam trawler built in 1900 by Hall Russell of Aberdeen.

The wreck charted at 560936N, 022600W was first reported in 1945. The position of the *Ben Attow* was given as 561130N, 022030W in 1968. Lloyds also give the same position, with the description 6 miles E by S of May Island, or 7 miles E $^1/_2$ S (note that E by S = 101.25°; E $^1/_2$ S = 95.625°). Seven miles E $^1/_2$ S is given in *British Vessels Lost at Sea 1939-1945*. 6 miles E by S results in a position of approximately 561100N, 022218W. Seven miles E $^1/_2$ S results in a position of approximately 561130N, 022042W.

These two positions are 1 mile apart, and both lie in an area within which no wrecks were found during a search by the Navy in 1977. 561130N, 022030W is also within that searched area, less than $^1/_2$ mile from 561130N, 022042W.

An unknown WW2 wreck is reported at 561000N, 022630W, which is 3.5 miles 120° from the May Island, and outside the searched area (not charted). The position recorded in 1945 at 560936N, 022600W, is $^1/_2$ mile further from the May, again outside the searched area. Yet another wreck position in the same general area was reported in 1955 at 560942N, 022115W, which is 6.5 miles 118° from the May (not charted). Could this be the *Ben Attow* (1940), *Thrive* (1946), *Eber* (1928) or another wreck?

SNELAND 1

Wreck No :	165	Date Sunk :	07 05 1945
Latitude :	56 09 40 N	Longitude :	02 30 48 W
Decca Lat :	5609.67 N	Decca Long :	0230.80 W
Location :	1.5 miles SE of May Island	Area :	May Island
Type :	Steamship	Tonnage :	1791 gross
Length :	320.1 feet Beam : 46.2 feet	Draught :	26.4 feet
How Sunk :	Torpedoed by U-2336	Depth :	44 metres

Sneland 1 (ex-*Ingeborg*), was a Norwegian steamship built in Stettin in 1922 by Nuscke & Co.

En route from Blyth for Belfast with 2800 tons of coal, she was torpedoed by U-2336 along with the *Avondale Park*, close by, in the last hour of WW2. Seven of the crew were lost out of a total of 26 crew plus 3 gunners.

Lloyds War Losses WW2, Vol. 1 gives position 560936N, 023124W for *Sneland 1*. In 1962, HMS *Scott* gave the position as 560940N, 023048W, and this is the charted position. *Dictionary of Disasters at Sea in the Age of Steam* gives the dimensions as 268 x 42.3 x 18 feet

UNKNOWN - EBER ?

Wreck No :	166	Date Sunk :	Pre-1955
Latitude :	56 09 42 N	Longitude :	02 21 15 W
Decca Lat :	5609.70 N	Decca Long :	0221.25 W
Location :	6.5 miles ESE of May Island	Area :	May Island
Type :		Tonnage :	
Length :	feet Beam : feet	Draught :	feet
How Sunk :		Depth :	58 metres

This wreck was first located in 1955 by HMS *Welcome*.

On 1st January 1928 the Leith-registered steam trawler *Eber* sprang a leak in heavy weather and foundered about 16 miles North of St. Abbs Head. The crew of seven took to their little boat, and after being buffeted for about two hours, were picked up in an exhausted condition by a passing steamer inward bound to the Forth.

The unknown wreck found at 560942N, 022115W in 1955 is about the right distance North of St. Abbs Head, and may be the *Eber*.

UB-63

Wreck No :	167	Date Sunk :	28 01 1918
Latitude :	56 10 00 N PA	Longitude :	02 00 00 W PA
Decca Lat :	5610.00 N	Decca Long :	0200.00 W
Location :	6.25 miles SE of May Island	Area :	May Island

Type :	Submarine	Tonnage :	508 gross
Length :	182.2 feet Beam : 18.9 feet	Draught :	feet
How Sunk :	D/C by HM Trawlers	Depth :	52 metres

UB-63 (Gebeschus) was a UBIII Class U-Boat built by Vulcan, Hamburg. This class was 508 tons surfaced, 639 tons submerged.

She was sunk by HM trawlers *W.S. Bailey* and *Fort George* on 20/1/1918.

See the wreck charted 8 miles 105° from S tip of May Island at 561010N, 021845W, which was first reported in this position on 24/3/1919.

UNKNOWN - PRE 1919

Wreck No :	168	Date Sunk :	Pre-1919
Latitude :	56 10 10 N	Longitude :	02 18 45 W
Decca Lat :	5610.17 N	Decca Long :	0218.75 W
Location :	8 miles 105° from May Island	Area :	May Island
Type :		Tonnage :	
Length :	feet Beam : feet	Draught :	feet
How Sunk :		Depth :	56 metres

A wreck was first reported in this position in 1919, but in 1977 the Navy found no trace of any wreck within a semicircle of radius 2.5 miles East through North to West of this position.

The wreck reported in 1919 may therefore lie slightly towards the South of this position, in the area not searched in 1977. Possibly the *UB-63* (1918)?

ASTA

Wreck No :	169	Date Sunk :	15 12 1927
Latitude :	56 10 11 N	Longitude :	02 21 34 W
Decca Lat :	5610.18 N	Decca Long :	0221.57 W
Location :	6¼ miles 105° from May Is.	Area :	May Island
Type :	Steamship	Tonnage :	1623 gross
Length :	254.0 feet Beam : 36.3 feet	Draught :	16.5 feet
How Sunk :	Collision with *Breslau*	Depth :	49 metres

The Swedish collier *Asta* (1623 tons, 254 x 36.3 x 16.5 feet) was en route from Methil to Copenhagen with a cargo of coal, when at 9.30 pm on Thursday 15th December 1927, about 8 miles East of the May Island, the steamship *Breslau* (1366 tons), belonging to James Currie & Co. of Leith, outward bound from Leith to Copenhagen with a general cargo, ran into her stern.

The *Asta*'s crew quickly realised their vessel was doomed and launched two of their boats. Within twenty minutes the *Asta* had sunk, and the crew of 19 were taken aboard the *Breslau*, which returned to Leith with damaged bows.

The wreck charted at 561011N, 022134W, 6.25 miles 105° from the May Island is apparently about 75 metres long (compared to 77 metres of the *Asta*). This position is shown on chart No. 175, published 9/12/1977. The position of this wreck was recorded as 561006N, 022132W in 1945.

UNKNOWN

Wreck No :	170		Date Sunk :	
Latitude :	56 10 11 N		Longitude :	02 32 37 W
Decca Lat :	5610.19 N		Decca Long :	0232.62 W
Location :	Off SW of May Island		Area :	May Island
Type :			Tonnage :	
Length :	feet	Beam : feet	Draught :	feet
How Sunk :			Depth :	54 metres

A wreck has been located and dived at Decca Red E16.76 - E16.80, Green F30.59 - F30.62, which converts to 561011N 023237W. The wreck is in 54 metres.

THRIVE

Wreck No :	171		Date Sunk :	20 02 1946
Latitude :	56 10 23 N		Longitude :	02 20 06 W
Decca Lat :	5610.38 N		Decca Long :	0220.10 W
Location :	7 miles 100° from May Island		Area :	May Island
Type :	Trawler		Tonnage :	
Length :	feet	Beam : feet	Draught :	feet
How Sunk :	Trawled up a mine		Depth :	58 metres

The *Thrive* sank when a mine exploded after being dragged up in her nets.

EMLEY

Wreck No :	172		Date Sunk :	28 04 1918
Latitude :	56 10 38 N		Longitude :	02 33 32 W
Decca Lat :	5610.63 N		Decca Long :	0233.52 W
Location :	3/4 mile 208° May Island Light		Area :	May Island
Type :	Trawler		Tonnage :	223 gross
Length :	112.1 feet	Beam : 22.5 feet	Draught :	12.5 feet
How Sunk :	Mined		Depth :	30 metres

The *Emley* was a steel screw ketch, (steam trawler), built in 1911 by Cochrane & Sons of Selby.

She was reported sunk by a mine on 28th April 1918 208° 3/4 mile from May Island light, and charted at 561030N, 023400W PA with at least 20 metres of water over it in general depths of 44 metres.

No wreck was located by HMS Scott in that position in 1959, but the wreck has since been located nearby at Decca Red E18.10, Green F32.13, which converts to 561039N, 023335W.

The charted position of the *Emley* has been altered to 561038N, 023332W in 30 metres.

PRIMROSE

Wreck No :	173	Date Sunk :	16 11 1904
Latitude :	56 10 42 N PA	Longitude :	02 33 21 W PA
Decca Lat :	5610.70 N	Decca Long :	0233.35 W
Location :	1/2 mile SW of May Island Light	Area :	May Island
Type :	Trawler	Tonnage :	91 gross
Length :	82.5 feet Beam : 18.0 feet	Draught :	8.0 feet
How Sunk :	Ran aground	Depth :	30 metres

In July 1992, Roy and Stuart Taylor of Fife Sub Aqua Club were dropped on a wreck which was initially supposed to be the *Emley*, but on recovering the bell, discovered that the wreck they were on was actually the *Primrose*, a steel-hulled Peterhead trawler which was reported lost by running aground on the South Ness of May Island on 16th November 1904 in a Force 6 South Westerly.

Primrose was a steel screw ketch (steam trawler), built in 1904 by Mackie & Thompson of Glasgow, engined by Ligerwood of Glasgow.

HOOSAC

Wreck No :	174	Date Sunk :	1926
Latitude :	56 10 30 N PA	Longitude :	02 33 30 W PA
Decca Lat :	5610.50 N	Decca Long :	0233.50 W
Location :	NE of Tarbet, May Island	Area :	May Island
Type :	Steamship	Tonnage :	5226 gross
Length :	400.0 feet Beam : 52.2 feet	Draught :	21.5 feet
How Sunk :	Not sunk	Depth :	metres

Hoosac (Ex-*Trojan Prince*, ex-*War Perch*), was built in 1918 by Bartram & Sons, Sunderland, engine by J. Dickinson & Sons, Sunderland. She was registered in Liverpool, and operated by Furness Withy. In 1926, Furness Lines sold four of their vessels, including *Hoosac*.

According to Les Pennington of *East Coast Divers*, whose information came from the May Island lighthouse keepers' logbook, the *Hoosac*, with a cargo of flour and grain, sank in 1926 North East of Tarbet, May Island.

No wreck is charted in that area, and there is no mention of the sinking of the *Hoosac* in the Scotsman newspaper in 1926.

The dimensions and tonnage of the *Hoosac* would make it one of the largest wrecks in the Forth, and one would have thought that it should be well documented.

The largest *Unknown* in the Forth appears to be the wreck 3.5 miles South of Elie at 560731N, 024904W, which sank pre - 1935, and I wondered if this might be the *Hoosac*, which does not appear in the 1927 *Lloyds Register*.

Unfortunately, the lighthouse keepers records for that period are no longer in existence, but enquiries to Lloyds brought forth the information that her name was changed to *Nemanja* by her new owners.

Whatever incident may have occurred off the May Island in 1926, she was not sunk then, but had a long life as the *Nemanja* until she was torpedoed and sunk on 7/4/1942 while carrying a cargo of 7207 tons of sugar on a voyage which left Maceris on 30/3/1942 to Halifax, Nova Scotia and the UK. Thirteen of her 47 crew were lost.

UNKNOWN - UB-63 ?

Wreck No :	175	Date Sunk :	Pre-03 1919
Latitude :	56 10 30 N PA	Longitude :	02 24 00 W PA
Decca Lat :	5610.50 N	Decca Long :	0224.00 W
Location :	5 miles 100° from May Island	Area :	May Island
Type :		Tonnage :	
Length :	feet Beam : feet	Draught :	feet
How Sunk :		Depth :	52 metres

A wreck was first reported in this charted PA on 24/3/1919.

See also *UB-63* at 561000N, 020000W PA, and *Unknown - pre-1919* at 561010N, 021845W.

GARIBALDI

Wreck No :	176	Date Sunk :	11 05 1870
Latitude :	56 10 50 N PA	Longitude :	02 32 30 W PA
Decca Lat :	5610.83 N	Decca Long :	0232.50 W
Location :	Off May Island	Area :	May Island
Type :	Paddle steamer	Tonnage :	73 gross
Length :	83.1 feet Beam : 17.9 feet	Draught :	9.1 feet
How Sunk :		Depth :	8 metres

Garibaldi was a wooden paddle steamer built in 1864, sunk off the May Island.

According to Brodie's *Steamers of the Forth*, she was a tug sunk while towing off North Berwick on 17th June 1870, yet later in the same book, she is said to have sunk off the May Island on 11/5/1870.

The Isle of May

The Isle of May

- 196
- Mars Rocks
- 198
- North Ness
- 193, 194, 195, 197
- N Horn
- Rona
- 178
- 184
- 188
- East Tarbet
- 182
- West Tarbet
- 183
- Altarstanes (West Landing)
- Tarbet Hole
- The Middens
- Low Light
- 185
- The Bishop
- Tower
- 170
- 181
- Kirk Haven
- The Pillow
- 177
- The Angel
- South Horn
- The Pilgrim
- The Cleaver
- Maiden Rocks
- Maiden Hair
- 173

N ↑

Chart showing the concentration of wrecks around the Isle of May. The popularity of hitting the northern rocks is apparent.

SCOTLAND

Wreck No : 177	Date Sunk : 19 03 1916
Latitude : 56 10 50 N PA	Longitude : 02 32 30 W PA
Decca Lat : 5610.83 N	Decca Long : 0232.50 W
Location : SE end, May Island	Area : May Island
Type : Steamship	Tonnage : 1490 gross
Length : 231.9 feet Beam : 35.7 feet	Draught : 22.9 feet
How Sunk : Ran aground	Depth : 8 metres

Scotland was a steel steamship with two decks, built in 1912 by Nylands of Christiania (Oslo), for Fred Olsen Lines, and registered in Norway.

She had a cargo of oak barrels, paper, and 3 motor boats at the time of running aground on the May Island while en route from Oslo to Grangemouth.

Strong tidal streams surround the May Island, and nowhere is this more evident than at the South end of the island, where the water flowing over the reef is very disturbed. As the island lies roughly North/South, and the tidal flow is East/West, the Northern and Southern extremities of the island are where the tidal streams are most noticeable. Off the West and the East of the island, the flow is almost imperceptible.

ALLOA

Wreck No : 178	Date Sunk : 02 01 1902
Latitude : 56 11 00 N PA	Longitude : 02 35 30 W PA
Decca Lat : 5611.00 N	Decca Long : 0235.50 W
Location : 4 miles SE of Anstruther	Area : May Island
Type : Steamship	Tonnage : 47 net
Length : feet Beam : feet	Draught : feet
How Sunk : Foundered	Depth : 25 metres

The position description is similar to that given by the *Footah* which sank after striking wreckage, presumably from the *Alloa*, on the same day. The net tonnage is 47, hence her gross tonnage is likely to be over 100.

AXEL

Wreck No : 179	Date Sunk : 18 10 1898
Latitude : 56 07 18 N PA	Longitude : 03 07 12 W PA
Decca Lat : 5607.30 N	Decca Long : 0307.20 W
Location : Harbour mouth, SE end, May Island	Area : May Island
Type : Barque	Tonnage : 520 gross
Length : feet Beam : feet	Draught : feet

How Sunk : Ran aground   Depth :   8 metres

Originally I believed that the Norwegian barque *Axel*, from London to Christiansand with a cargo of coke, was blown on to the rocks of the May Island, near the harbour mouth, in an Easterly storm Force 10, on 18th October 1898.

However, I have now discovered that the *Axel* of Frederickstadt, was driven ashore at Dysart in an Easterly storm Force 10 on 18th October 1898. Between 3 am and 4 am she was sighted by the coastguard station, drifting helplessly before the wind. Her rudder was evidently disabled and she had become unmanageable. In about half an hour she was dashed on the rocks between the Noop and the harbour. The crew of 10 were all saved. The rock on which she was driven was shattered by the impact, and her hull was seriously damaged.

The *Axel* had left London about a fortnight previously for Christiansand with a cargo of 509 tons of coke. She experienced terribly stormy weather in the North Sea, and made for the Forth for shelter.

A large number of people visited the scene of the wreck during the day and several even clambered aboard to assist in cutting away the mast. The grog keg was broached, with the result that one man had to be taken home in a cart, along with the boxes, ropes, etc. saved from the wreck.

DUNBRITTON

Wreck No : 180   Date Sunk : 03 02 1906
Latitude :   56 11 00 N PA   Longitude : 02 33 00 W PA
Decca Lat : 5611.00 N   Decca Long : 0233.00 W
Location :   Off May Island   Area :   May Island
Type :   Iron Barque   Tonnage :   1536 gross
Length :   234.3 feet   Beam : 39.6 feet Draught :   23.1 feet
How Sunk :   Depth :   metres

According to Les Pennington, the 1536 ton iron barque *Dunbritton* sank off May Island on 3rd February 1906, but a report in the *Scotsman* newspaper of Monday 5th February tells a different story.

The Glasgow barque *Dunbritton* had left Hamburg for Honolulu with a general cargo, but sustained so much damage in stormy conditions in the North Sea that she had to run to Leith for repairs. She left that port to resume her voyage on 25th January, and by that afternoon had scarcely made Fair Isle (this must be a misprint for May Isle as it would have been quite impossible for to have covered anything like the distance of over 300 miles to Fair Isle in only a few hours) when she again encountered SW gales and very heavy seas. Her foremast and mizzen topmast were carried away, and she was blown for 35 miles before her uncontrolled drift could be arrested. The wind veered to NW with snow storms, then backed to SW then WSW.

The vessel was obviously in very serious difficulties by then, and was taken in tow by the Hull trawler *Mary Stuart*. For three days, during which the intensity of the storm increased, the trawler attempted to reach the Firth of Forth. The tow finally had to be slipped when the *Dunbritton*'s main mast was brought down by the force of the storm and her deck was damaged allowing water to enter the ship at a greater rate than her pumps could cope with.

A second trawler, the *Loch Stenness*, appeared on the scene, and both trawlers took the gradually sinking *Dunbritton* in tow for a time until this had to be abandoned at about 5530N 0020E. The crew of the barque used their own lifeboat to transfer to the *Loch Stenness*, and their own vessel was soon lost to sight, and is presumed to have foundered shortly thereafter. The *Loch Stenness* landed the barque's crew at Aberdeen on Sunday 4th February.

ISLAND

Wreck No :	181	Date Sunk :	13 04 1937
Latitude :	56 11 02 N	Longitude :	02 32 52 W
Decca Lat :	5611.03 N	Decca Long :	0232.87 W
Location :	ESE of May Island Tower	Area :	May Island
Type :	Steamship	Tonnage :	1774 gross
Length :	250.0 feet Beam : 40.0 feet	Draught :	feet
How Sunk :	Ran aground	Depth :	13 metres

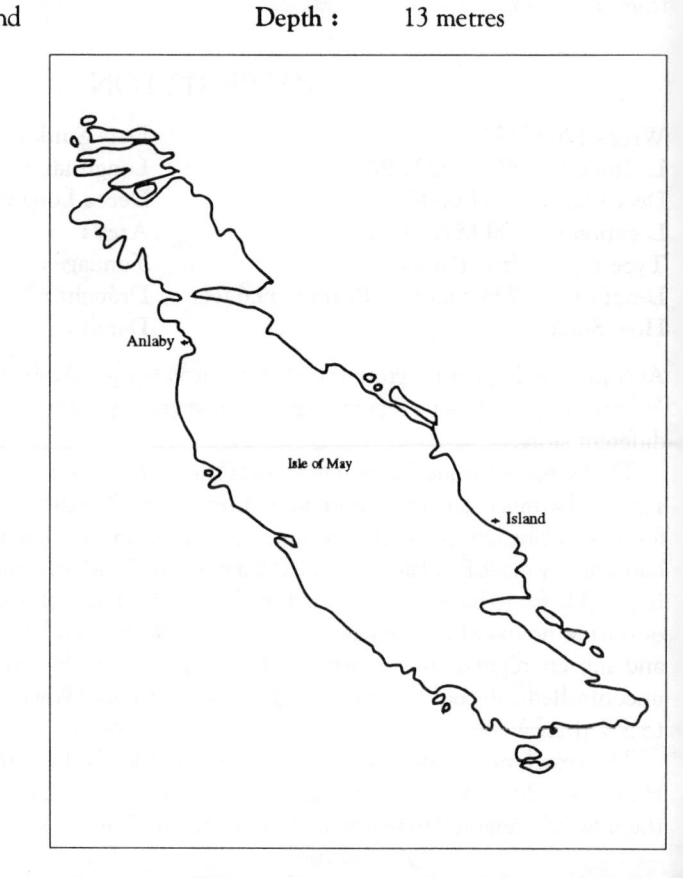

The sites of the wrecks of the Island and the Anlaby on the Isle of May

The 1774 ton steamship *Island*, formerly the Danish Royal Yacht, bound from Copenhagen to Leith, ran on to the East side of the May in dense fog.

Because of the fog the light could not be seen, and the foghorn signal was heard only twice before the vessel struck the rocks.

Parts of the wreck are visible on the rocks on the East of the May Island, 1/4 mile from the lighthouse.

JASPER

Wreck No :	182	Date Sunk :	17 04 1894
Latitude :	56 11 12 N PA	Longitude :	02 33 03 W PA
Decca Lat :	5611.20 N	Decca Long :	0233.05 W
Location :	500 yards SE by E May Island Light	Area :	May Island
Type :	Steamship	Tonnage :	1256 gross
Length :	235.0 feet Beam : 31.7 feet	Draught :	22.4 feet
How Sunk :	Ran aground	Depth :	8 metres

The British steamship *Jasper*, built in 1883 by W.B. Thompson, was wrecked on May Island on 17th April 1894, while en route from Dundee to Burntisland in ballast. The ship was 811 tons net.

LINNET

Wreck No :	183	Date Sunk :	07 08 1877
Latitude :	56 11 12 N PA	Longitude :	02 33 00 W PA
Decca Lat :	5611.20 N	Decca Long :	0233.00 W
Location :	E. side of May Island	Area :	May Island
Type :	Schooner	Tonnage :	97 gross
Length :	feet Beam : feet	Draught :	feet
How Sunk :	Ran aground	Depth :	20 metres

The Aberdeen schooner *Linnet* ran on to the East side of the May Island while bound from Newburgh to Sunderland with a cargo of oats on 7th August 1877.

ANLABY

Wreck No :	184	Date Sunk :	23 08 1873
Latitude :	56 11 15 N	Longitude :	02 33 52 W
Decca Lat :	5611.25 N	Decca Long :	0233.87 W
Location :	N of West Landing, May Island	Area :	May Island

Type :	Steamship		Tonnage :	1110 gross	
Length :	231.0 feet	Beam : 32.0 feet	Draught :	17.0 feet	
How Sunk :	Ran aground		Depth :	20 metres	

The steamship *Anlaby*, with a cargo of coal, ran into the rocks North of the West Landing, May Island on 23rd August 1873.

A report in the *Fife Free Press* of Saturday 30th August 1873 names the vessel as the *Plaby* of Hull but this must be a phonetic error. Anlaby is the name of an area on the outskirts of Hull. She had left Granton bound for Danzig with coal, and was proceeding dead slow in fog. At about 6 pm she went on to the rocks on the West side of the May Island, with her forefoot on the rock and her stern in 8 fathoms (15 metres) of water. Lighters and a tug were sent to her assistance but failed to take her off.

All that remains are iron ribs of the keel, and a large 4-bladed iron propeller. She lies E/W with her bows pointing towards the May Island.

CARMEN OF STOCKHOLM

Wreck No :	185	Date Sunk :	20 01 1923	
Latitude :	56 11 18 N PA	Longitude :	02 33 15 W PA	
Decca Lat :	5611.30 N	Decca Long :	0233.25 W	
Location :	200 yards W of May Island Light	Area :	May Island	
Type :	Schooner	Tonnage :	1590 gross	
Length :	feet Beam : feet	Draught :	feet	
How Sunk :	Ran aground	Depth :	22 metres	

According to Les Pennington of East Coast Divers, the schooner *Carmen of Stockholm* was lost 200 yards West of the May Island light in 1923.

On investigation, however, the truth turned out to be very different. To avoid others in the future needlessly looking for this wreck, I include the following information from the *Fife Free Press* of Saturday 20th January 1923.

The schooner *Carmen*, a four-masted motor vessel belonging to Stockholm, ran ashore 800 yards West of Fife Ness Point, near Crail, early on Saturday morning, 13th January. The *Carmen* had left South Shields after discharging a cargo of pit props, and was proceeding light to Grangemouth to load a cargo of coal for Barcelona. A dense fog overhung the Forth during the night, and it appears that the captain, who was part owner of the vessel, missed direction while attempting to enter the Forth. The vessel struck the rocks at 5.45 am and, at 5.50 am, fired a flare. The watchman at the Fife Ness Coastguard station had, however, already observed the schooner. The life-saving apparatus was called out immediately and was used to save the crew. The local lifeboat was also launched and stood by the vessel.

During the day, a salvage tug from Leith arrived and, by midnight, had succeeded in dragging the vessel from the rocks into a good position. A second tug was summoned and the *Carmen* was successfully towed to Leith for repairs.

NEWCASTLE PACKET

Wreck No :	186	Date Sunk :	02 04 1889
Latitude :	56 11 20 N	Longitude :	02 33 00 W
Decca Lat :	5611.33 N	Decca Long :	0233.00 W
Location :	Stranded May Island	Area :	May Island
Type :	Schooner	Tonnage :	72 gross
Length :	feet Beam : feet	Draught :	feet
How Sunk :	Ran aground	Depth :	metres

The Norwegian schooner *Newcastle Packet* had a cargo of firewood from Christiansand to Grangemouth when she ran on to the May Island in a Force 6 North Easterly wind.

She will therefore be lying somewhere along the East side of the May.

CARL KONOW

Wreck No :	187	Date Sunk :	1883
Latitude :	56 11 25 N PA	Longitude :	02 34 00 W PA
Decca Lat :	5611.42 N	Decca Long :	0234.00 W
Location :	NW of May Island Light	Area :	May Island
Type :	Steamship	Tonnage :	300 gross
Length :	feet Beam : feet	Draught :	feet
How Sunk :		Depth :	27 metres

According to Les Pennington of East Coast Divers, the 300 ton steamship *Carl Konow* was in ballast at the time of loss North West of the May Island light in 1883, but there is no mention of that vessel in the 1883 editions of the *Fife Free Press* or the *Fifeshire Advertiser*, nor in contemporary *Parliamentary Papers*, or *Lloyds Register of Shipping*! Did she exist?

In fact, 1883 was a year of extremely bad weather, and as a result, quite a number of vessels were lost that year.

Her name suggests she was not a British vessel, and if she was overcome by stress of weather and foundered with all hands while outward bound to a foreign port, it may have been some time before she was missed due to non-arrival at her destination. That may account for the lack of information in the newspapers of the time. Also in those days, registration with *Lloyds* was probably only voluntary, for insurance purposes, and that may account for her non-appearance in *Lloyds Register*.

KATRINE

Wreck No :	188	Date Sunk :	1871
Latitude :	56 11 25 N	Longitude :	02 33 30 W
Decca Lat :	5611.42 N	Decca Long :	0233.50 W
Location :	Mouth of Tarbet, E. side May Is.	Area :	May Island

Type :	Steamship			Tonnage :	280 gross
Length :	feet	Beam :	feet	Draught :	feet
How Sunk :	Ran aground?			Depth :	30 metres

Katrine had a cargo of iron plates.

DURHAM COAST

Wreck No :	189			Date Sunk :	1926
Latitude :	56 11 30 N PA			Longitude :	02 33 30 W PA
Decca Lat :	5611.50 N			Decca Long :	0233.50 W
Location :	near May Island			Area :	May Island
Type :	Steamship			Tonnage :	783 gross
Length :	215.0 feet	Beam :	32.0 feet	Draught :	12.3 feet
How Sunk :	Not sunk			Depth :	metres

According to East Coast Divers guide to the Forth, the wreck of the steamship *Durham Coast* lies "near the May Island".

There are a number of *Unknowns* in the vicinity of the May Island, but the *Durham Coast* is not one of them.

She was a steel screw steamship built in 1912 by Goole S.B. Co., engine by Richardsons, Westgarth & Co., Middlesbrough, registered in Liverpool and owned by Coast Lines.

The report of her loss near the May Island in 1926 was greatly exaggerated, as in 1948 her name was changed to *Rama-Raja*, and she was eventually broken up in India in 1957.

UNKNOWN

Wreck No :	190			Date Sunk :	
Latitude :	56 11 30 N PA			Longitude :	02 11 30 W PA
Decca Lat :	5611.50 N			Decca Long :	0211.50 W
Location :	12 miles E of May Island			Area :	May Island
Type :				Tonnage :	
Length :	feet	Beam :	feet	Draught :	feet
How Sunk :				Depth :	49 metres

An unknown wreck is charted at 561130N, 021130W PA with at least 49 metres over it in about 59 metres, 12 miles East of the May Island.

UNKNOWN - MALLARD ?

Wreck No :	191	Date Sunk :	
Latitude :	56 11 30 N PA	Longitude :	02 28 30 W PA
Decca Lat :	5611.50 N	Decca Long :	0228.50 W
Location :	2.5 miles E of May Island	Area :	May Island
Type :		Tonnage :	
Length : feet	Beam : feet	Draught :	feet
How Sunk :		Depth :	52 metres

The wreck charted at 561130N, 022830W PA within the disused ammunition and boom gear dumping ground East of May Island, is recorded by the Hydrographic Department as the steamship *Mallard*, sunk in 1921.

There does not seem to be any record of a wreck having been found here during any of the surveys which have been carried out, and this appears to be only a convenient approximate position to represent the loss of the *Mallard* near the May Island, and may not necessarily imply that there is actually any wreck in, or close to, that position.

HILDA

Wreck No :	192	Date Sunk :	29 08 1939
Latitude :	56 11 33 N PA	Longitude :	02 33 30 W PA
Decca Lat :	5611.55 N	Decca Long :	0233.50 W
Location :	E. side of N. Ness, May Island	Area :	May Island
Type :	Steamship	Tonnage :	643 gross
Length : feet	Beam : feet	Draught :	feet
How Sunk :	Ran aground/refloated	Depth :	metres

The 643 tons gross steamship *Hilda*, en route from Rauma Luvia, Finland to Leith with a cargo of 630 standards of wood, ran on to the East side of the North Ness, May Island at 2.20 am on 29th August, 1939.

She had been entering the Forth by the North channel between Fife and the May Island in thick fog. The May Island fog signal was heard and recognised, but was thought to be more distant than it really was. The vessel was holed on the port side about one third of her length from the bow and the forward hold was flooded. A tug and the Anstruther lifeboat stood by, and as the weather was calm with little swell, the 17 crew remained aboard in the hope that their vessel could be refloated at high tide. This subsequently proved to be the case, and after being refloated, she proceeded up the Firth of Forth towards Leith.

The lighthouse keeper's report does not say whether this was under her own power or in tow by the tug, nor is it known whether she arrived at Leith or sank en route to that port.

LOUISE HENRIETTA

Wreck No :	193	Date Sunk :	
Latitude :	56 11 33 N PA	Longitude :	02 33 30 W PA
Decca Lat :	5611.55 N	Decca Long :	0233.50 W
Location :	E. side of N. Ness, May Island	Area :	May Island
Type :	Schooner	Tonnage :	209 gross
Length :	feet Beam : feet	Draught :	feet
How Sunk :	Ran aground	Depth :	8 metres

The schooner *Louise Henrietta* had a cargo of railway sleepers.

GEORGE AUNGER

Wreck No :	194	Date Sunk :	25 04 1930
Latitude :	56 11 33 N PA	Longitude :	02 33 30 W PA
Decca Lat :	5611.55 N	Decca Long :	0233.50 W
Location :	E. side of N. Ness, May Island	Area :	May Island
Type :	Trawler	Tonnage :	273 gross
Length :	125.4 feet Beam : 22.7 feet	Draught :	12.2 feet
How Sunk :	Ran aground	Depth :	8 metres

The 273 ton steam trawler *George Aunger*, built in 1918 by Cook, Welton & Gemmell of Beverley, Hull, and belonging to G.W. & J. Leiper of Aberdeen went ashore at 11.10 pm on 25th April 1930 in thick fog on the East side of North Ness, May Island.

Although the fog signal had been heard, it was thought to be 3 or 4 miles distant. In the high seas running, her skipper and fireman were washed overboard and lost, D. Morris, the skipper being swept out through the wheel house window. The four other crew members were rescued by the lighthouse keepers who displayed great gallantry in climbing aboard the trawler by the anchor chain at low tide, some time after the vessel struck.

The Anstruther and Broughty Ferry lifeboats were called to the scene, but owing to the heavy seas were unable to render assistance. One of the Anstruther lifeboatmen expressed the opinion that no lifeboat ever built could have assisted in the prevailing conditions. The lighthouse keepers carried the survivors across the island to the more sheltered West side, where they were transferred to the waiting lifeboat.

VICTORY

Wreck No :	195	Date Sunk :	06 03 1934
Latitude :	56 11 33 N PA	Longitude :	02 33 30 W PA
Decca Lat :	5611.55 N	Decca Long :	0233.50 W
Location :	Norman Rock, N. Ness, May Island	Area :	May Island

Type :	Trawler		Tonnage :	164 gross	
Length :	102.3 feet	Beam : 19.8 feet	Draught :	10.0 feet	
How Sunk :	Ran aground		Depth :	8 metres	

The iron-hulled Aberdeen steam trawler *Victory* (A 692), 164 tons, built in 1898, went on the rocks at the North Ness of May Island at 8.20 pm on 6th March 1934. All on board were saved.

In his book about Aberdenn steam trawler losses, *The Real Price of Fish*, George F. Ritchie states that the *Victory* was on a coaling trip to the Forth with a crew of nine. At 8.00 pm in dense fog, she ran aground at the North end of the May Isle. She was badly damaged and filled with water within two hours. Anstruther lifeboat set out in response to her distress flares and siren sounding, but before the lifeboat arrived at the scene, in spite of a choppy sea, the Anstruther fishing boat *Enterprise* had already succeeded in getting near enough the wreck to take off the nine crewmen.

This account is at variance with the lighthouse keepers report which says the *Victory* went aground on the North Ness at 8.20 pm in clear weather, wind Westerly Force 3. There was only a slight swell. The May Island light was on, but the fog signal was not sounding. (Because there was no fog!).

THOMAS L. DEVLIN

Wreck No : 196
Latitude : 56 11 33 N

Date Sunk : 20 12 1959
Longitude : 02 33 54 W

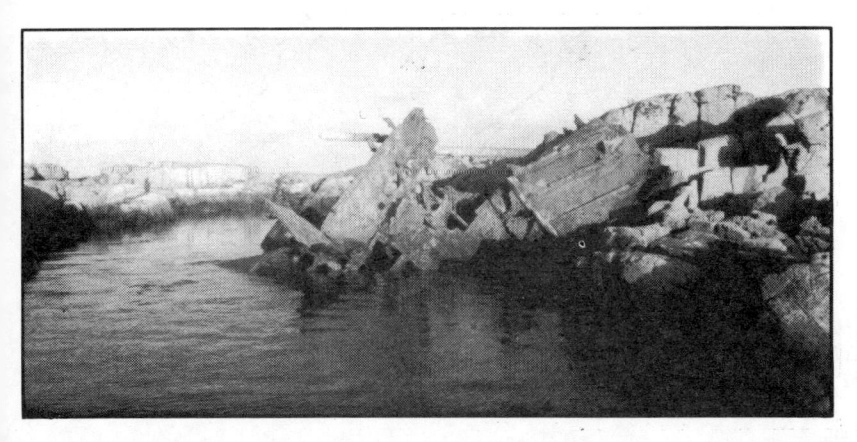

The remains of the Thomas L. Devlin on the North Ness of the Isle of May. Photo by Bob Baird.

Decca Lat:	5611.55 N	**Decca Long:**	0233.90 W
Location:	North Ness, May Island	**Area:**	May Island
Type:	Trawler	**Tonnage:**	211 gross
Length:	115.7 feet **Beam:** 22.6 feet	**Draught:**	12.2 feet
How Sunk:	Ran aground	**Depth:**	18 metres

The Granton trawler *Thomas L Devlin* (ex-*Phyllis Belman*), was built in 1915 by A. Hall & Co. of Aberdeen.

She ran on to the North Ness of May Island at 9.15 pm on 20th December 1959 in clear weather. Her 13 crew were rescued by the Anstruther lifeboat.

A large chunk of rusty steel wreckage lies above water, wedged in the inlet between North Ness and Mars Rock. Is this part of the *Thomas L Devlin*?

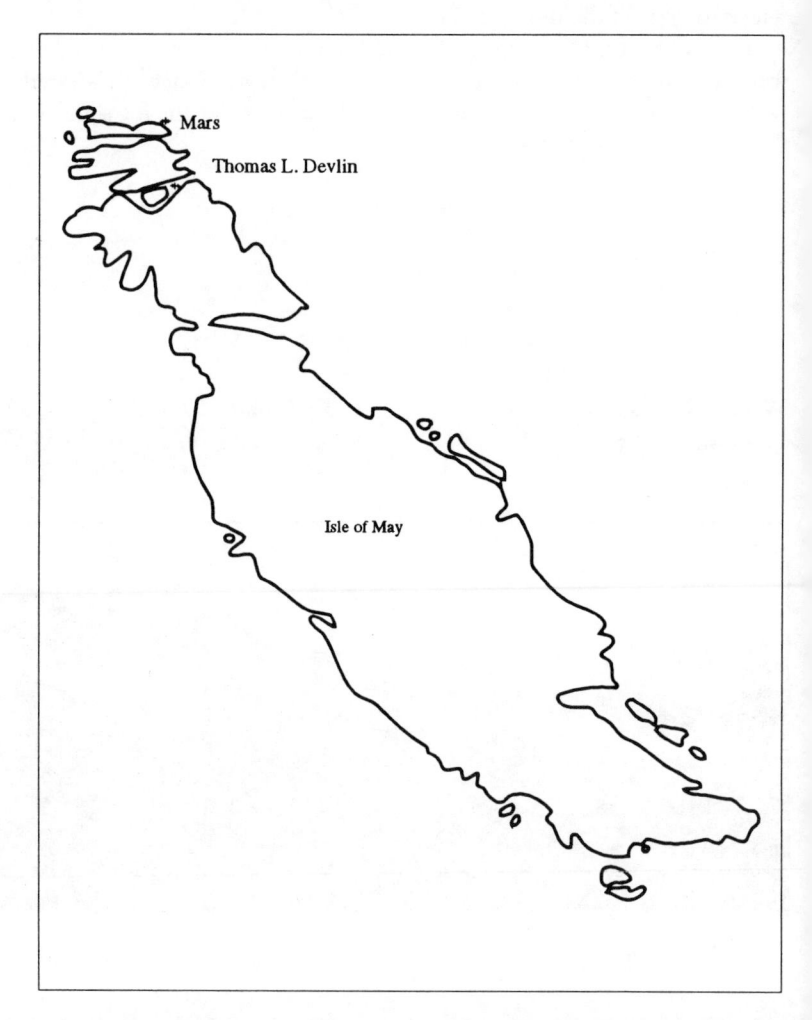

Sites of the wrecks of the Thomas L. Devlin and the Mars on the North east of the Isle of May near North Ness

MATA GARDA

Wreck No :	197	Date Sunk :	1872
Latitude :	56 11 33 N PA	Longitude :	02 33 30 W PA
Decca Lat :	5611.55 N	Decca Long :	0233.50 W
Location :	E. side of N. Ness, May Island	Area :	May Island
Type :	Schooner	Tonnage :	153 gross
Length : feet Beam : feet		Draught :	feet
How Sunk :		Depth :	8 metres

The 3-masted schooner *Mata Garda* had a cargo of coal.

MARS

Wreck No :	198	Date Sunk :	19 05 1936
Latitude :	56 11 35 N	Longitude :	02 33 52 W
Decca Lat :	5611.58 N	Decca Long :	0233.87 W
Location :	Mars Rock, N. Ness, may island	Area :	May Island
Type :	Steamship	Tonnage :	540 gross
Length : feet Beam : feet		Draught :	feet
How Sunk :	Ran aground	Depth :	18 metres

The Latvian steamship *Mars*, bound from Ireland to Methil, ran on to the North Ness of May Island at 2.15 am on 19th May 1936 while entering the Firth of Forth in fog. Although the fog signal was sounding, it was not heard. The 13 crew were all saved.

MALLARD

Wreck No :	199	Date Sunk :	13 07 1921
Latitude :	56 11 49 N	Longitude :	02 35 25 W
Decca Lat :	5611.82 N	Decca Long :	0235.42 W
Location :	1 mile WNW of May Island	Area :	May Island
Type :	Steamship	Tonnage :	213 gross
Length :	125.8 feet Beam : 23.6 feet	Draught :	12.1 feet
How Sunk :	Foundered	Depth :	42 metres

This wreck was located by HNLMS *Alkmaar* during an exercise in February 1989. She lies N/S with bow pointing North, length 40 metres, beam 9 metres, has a bridge aft, and a large single hold amidships.

This description seems to suggest a small steamship with well deck forward, and machinery aft - a very common configuration. Decca Red E22.50, Green F36.30, 1 mile

300°. from May Island.

It is not charted yet, but C. Aspinall and R. Taylor of Fife Sub Aqua Club dived this wreck in 1990, and reported an iron or steel ship similar to a puffer, sitting upright and apparently intact, with no obvious indication of the reason for sinking. The hold is full of coal, and the wreck appeared to have been on the sand and shingle bottom for some considerable time. Two portholes and the steam whistle were recovered, but no items to aid identification. The recovered items were lying loose, having become detached from their fastenings by long immersion.

The *Alloa* and the *Footah* sank in this vicinity in 1902, but this wreck seems to be larger than either of these two vessels.

The most likely possibility is the steamship *Mallard*, built in 1875 by Earles of Hull. She foundered en route from Dysart to Aberdeen with a cargo of coal. The vessel was caught in a heavy wind in the Firth of Forth, and the crew were helpless until the arrival of the motor boat *Baldie Snowdrop*, which took them off and landed them safely in Anstruther.

FOOTAH

Wreck No : 200
Latitude : 56 12 00 N PA
Decca Lat : 5612.00 N
Location : 4 miles SE by E of Anstruther
Type : Steamship
Length : 95.1 feet Beam : 14.2 feet
How Sunk : Struck wreckage

Date Sunk : 02 01 1902
Longitude : 02 35 00 W PA
Decca Long : 0235.00 W
Area : May Island
Tonnage : 100 gross
Draught : 8.7 feet
Depth : 25 metres

The Alloa-registered iron steamship *Footah* struck wreckage and sank 4 miles SE by E of Anstruther on 2nd January 1902. The wreckage struck was presumably from the *Alloa*, which foundered nearby on the same day.

Footah was 47 tons net, built in 1884 by Jones of Liverpool and registered in Barrow.

UNKNOWN - PRE 1919

Wreck No : 201
Latitude : 56 12 20 N PA
Decca Lat : 5612.33 N
Location : 1 mile NE of May Island
Type :
Length : feet Beam : feet
How Sunk :

Date Sunk : Pre-03 1919
Longitude : 02 33 10 W PA
Decca Long : 0233.17 W
Area : May Island
Tonnage :
Draught : feet
Depth : 40 metres

The wreck charted one mile North East of May Island at 561220N, 023310W PA with at least 28 metres over it in 45 metres, was reported on 24 March 1919. Decca co-ordinates for this wreck are Red E22.57, Green F36.77.19.

The *Northumbria* sank a mile from this PA in 1917, and this may be a slightly incorrect estimate of the position of the wreck of the *Northumbria*.

Many vessels are known to have been lost near the May Island over the years, and this may be the position of one of the vessels named elsewhere in this book for which no accurate position has yet been established.

It is, of course, also possible that this may be another wreck altogether. One possibility is that this may be the bows of the *K-14*, which were sheared off in collision with the *K-22* during the Battle of May Island on 31st January 1918. Another possibility is that this may be the sloop *Packet*, with a cargo of coal. She was reported sunk half a mile North East of the May Island in 1817.

NORTHUMBRIA

Wreck No :	202	Date Sunk :	03 03 1917
Latitude :	56 12 26 N	Longitude :	02 34 43 W
Decca Lat :	5612.43 N	Decca Long :	0234.72 W
Location :	1 mile N of May Island	Area :	May Island
Type :	Trawler	Tonnage :	211 gross
Length :	115.5 feet Beam : 19.8 feet	Draught :	9.9 feet
How Sunk :	Mined	Depth :	33 metres

The 211 ton steam trawler *Northumbria* was mined one mile North of the May Island on 3rd March 1917, and now lies at 561226N, 023443W.

The boiler stands 4 metres high, but the remainder of the wreckage is no more than 1 metre high in a general depth of 34 metres.

Decca co-ordinates: Red E 22.48, Green F 36.75 (given in 1987), and Red E 22.52, Green F 36.85 (Colin Aspinall 1989).

See the wreck charted at 561220N, 023310W PA, first reported 24/3/1919.

UNKNOWN - WW2 ?

Wreck No :	203	Date Sunk :	WW2
Latitude :	56 12 30 N PA	Longitude :	02 27 00 W PA
Decca Lat :	5612.50 N	Decca Long :	0227.00 W
Location :	3.75 miles E of May Island	Area :	May Island
Type :		Tonnage :	
Length :	feet Beam : feet	Draught :	feet

How Sunk :   **Depth :**   52 metres

The wreck charted as Wk PA at 561230N, 022700W, 3.75 miles East of the May Island was reported in 1945, and is thought to be an unknown WW2 loss.

UNKNOWN - BEN ATTOW ?

Wreck No :	204		**Date Sunk :**		
Latitude :	56 12 49 N		**Longitude :**	02 24 58 W	
Decca Lat :	5612.82 N		**Decca Long :**	0224.97 W	
Location :	5 miles E of May Island		**Area :**	May Island	
Type :			**Tonnage :**		
Length :	100.0 feet	**Beam :** feet	**Draught :**		feet
How Sunk :			**Depth :**	52 metres	

The wreck charted at 561249N, 022458W in a depth of 52 metres 5 miles East of the May Island is apparently 100 feet long. This may possibly be the *Ben Attow*.

UNKNOWN - BALLOCHBUIE ?

Wreck No :	205		**Date Sunk :**	Pre-1962	
Latitude :	56 13 41 N		**Longitude :**	02 14 00 W	
Decca Lat :	5613.68 N		**Decca Long :**	0214.00 W	
Location :	11 miles E of May Island		**Area :**	May Island	
Type :			**Tonnage :**		
Length :	200.0 feet	**Beam :** feet	**Draught :**		feet
How Sunk :			**Depth :**	45 metres	

The wreck charted at 561341N, 021400W, 11 miles East of the May Island was first located in 1962 by *HMS Scott*. The least depth was reported as 45 metres, and the wreck was standing up some 8.5 metres from the sea bed which is at 54 metres. This wreck is apparently 200 feet long, which coincides with the length of the *Ballochbuie*.

QUEENSLAND ?

Wreck No :	206		**Date Sunk :**	14 02 1883
Latitude :	56 13 42 N		**Longitude :**	02 24 12 W
Decca Lat :	5613.70 N		**Decca Long :**	0224.20 W
Location :	6 miles E of May Island		**Area :**	May Island

THE ISLE OF MAY

Type : Lugsailer　　　　　　　Tonnage : 34 gross
Length : 　　feet　Beam : 　　feet　Draught : 　　feet
How Sunk : Foundered　　　　　Depth : 55 metres

A wreck is charted at 561342N, 022412W, 6 miles East of the May Island, in 55 metres of water. This may be the 34 ton lugsailer *Queensland* which was reported to have foundered 7 miles E of May Island.

The crew of the Prestonpans fishing boat *Queensland* were hauling in their lines when the boat shipped a heavy sea which threw her on her beam ends and capsized her, with the loss of all 7 of the crew. According to the crews of two other Prestonpans fishing boats, *Delight* and *Blue Jack*, who witnessed it, the disaster took place about 20 miles East of the May Island. Because of the heavy sea, the horrified watchers were unable to render assistance.

BALLOCHBUIE ?

Wreck No : 207　　　　　　　　Date Sunk : 20 04 1917
Latitude : 56 13 46 N　　　　　 Longitude : 02 23 36 W
Decca Lat : 5613.77 N　　　　　Decca Long : 0223.60 W
Location : 6 miles E of May Island　Area : May Island
Type : Steamship　　　　　　　Tonnage : 921 gross
Length : 200.0 feet　Beam : 31.3 feet　Draught : 12.7 feet
How Sunk : Torpedoed　　　　　Depth : 53 metres

Ballochbuie was a 921 ton steel screw steamship built in 1905 by John Duthie S.B. Co., Aberdeen, engine by J. Abernethy, Aberdeen, and registered in Aberdeen.

When she was torpedoed on 20th April 1917, the master and two of the crew were lost. In 1968 the Navy gave the position 561300N, 021800W, 9 miles E of May Island. *Lloyds* gives 7 miles E of May Island. The nearest charted wreck is at 561346N, 022336W, 6 miles East of May Island.

K-17

Wreck No : 208　　　　　　　　Date Sunk : 31 01 1918
Latitude : 56 15 21 N　　　　　 Longitude : 02 11 41 W
Decca Lat : 5615.35 N　　　　　Decca Long : 0211.68 W
Location : 13 miles E of Fife Ness　Area : May Island
Type : Submarine　　　　　　　Tonnage : 2565 gross
Length : 338.0 feet　Beam : 　26.6 feet　Draught : 　　feet
How Sunk : Collision with *Fearless*　Depth : 46 metres

First located by HMS *Scott* in 1962. Least depth 46 metres and standing up some 6 metres from the seabed at 51 metres.

K-17 was sunk in collision with HMS *Fearless*.

K-4

Wreck No :	209	Date Sunk :	31 01 1918
Latitude :	56 15 32 N	Longitude :	02 11 00 W
Decca Lat :	5615.53 N	Decca Long :	0211.40 W
Location :	13 miles E of Fife Ness	Area :	May Island
Type :	Submarine	Tonnage :	2565 gross
Length :	338.0 feet Beam : 26.6 feet	Draught :	feet
How Sunk :	Collision with K-6	Depth :	46 metres

First located by HMS Scott in 1962. Least depth 46 metres and standing up some 7 metres from the sea bed at 53 metres.

The K-4 was sunk in collision with HM submarine K-6. As she turned over when sinking, the K-4 is possibly lying upside down. If this is the case, even had she been fitted with escape apparatus, it would probably have been useless.

NOTE: *Some of the wrecks listed in this book may be considered to be War Graves - notably K-4 and HMS Pathfinder. War Graves are covered by the Protection of Military Remains Act 1986 and include the wrecks of any Royal Navy ship or merchant vessel lost on active Government service and which have human remains aboard. Apparently it is normally permissible to dive on these wrecks but not to disturb or remove anything from the site.*

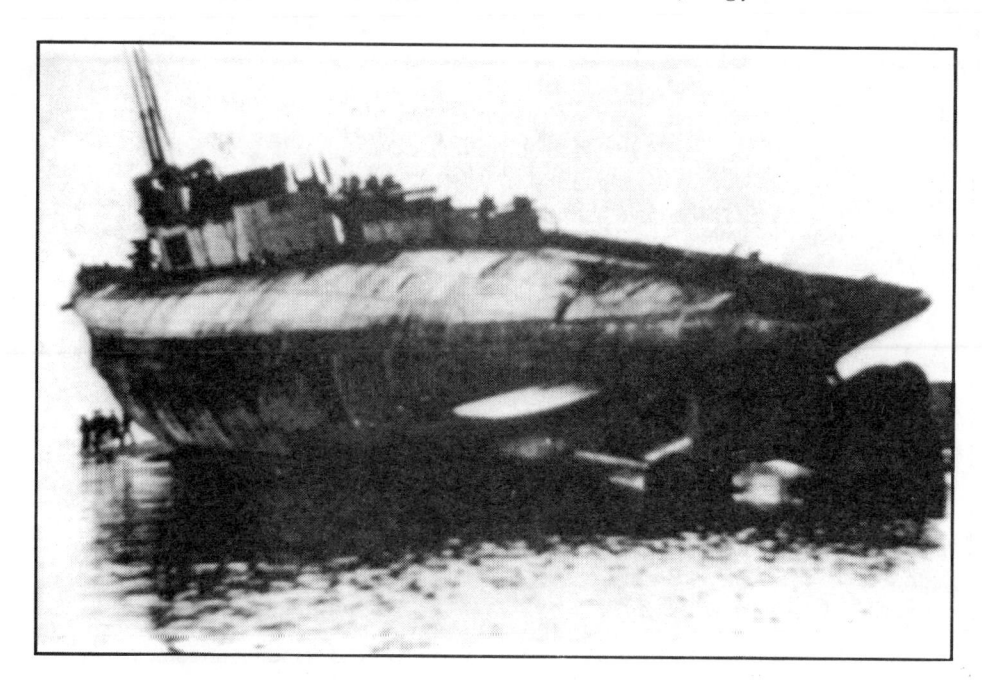

Below: K-4 aground on Walney Island during her trials off Barrow in Furness. Photograph Mirrorpic.

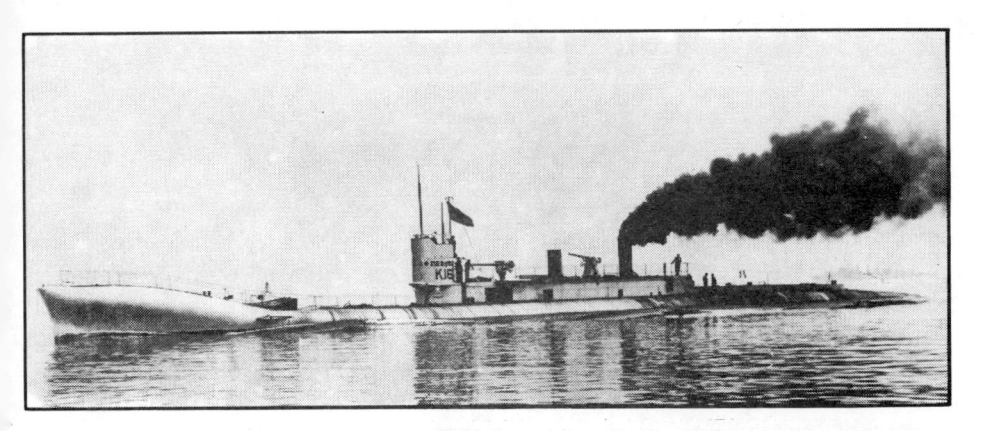

Above: K-16, sister vessel of K-4 and K-17, both lost in the Forth. (Photograph courtesy of Ian Johnson)

Below: K-6 before the bulbous bow was fitted. (Photograph courtesy of the Imperial War Museum.)

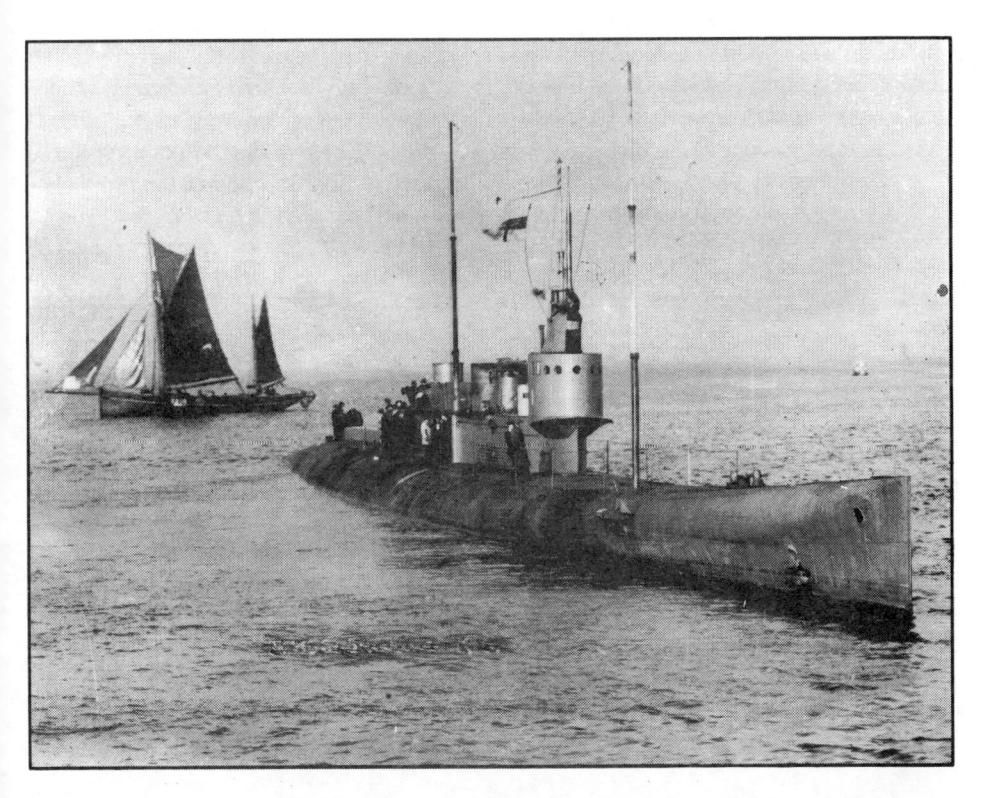

The Battle of May Island

The sinking of HM Submarines K-4 and K-17

THE SUBMARINES. The K Class submarines were monsters in their day, being twice as long and three times as heavy as other submarines of that era, and had no fewer than seven power sources driving their twin propellers - two steam turbines of 10500 shp gave a maximum speed of 24 knots on the surface, four electric motors of 1400 hp which produced a maximum speed underwater of 9 knots, and an auxiliary diesel engine of 1800 hp for manoeuvring on the surface while building up steam. Their normal complement was 53 men, and the maximum diving depth was 150 feet The armament consisted of ten 18" torpedo tubes, two of which were mounted in the funnel superstructure for surface use at night, two 4-inch guns, (except K-17 which had 5.5-inch guns), and one 3-inch anti-aircraft gun

Because of their technical complexity, a time-consuming procedure had to be carried out before diving. This included extinguishing the boiler furnaces for steam production, retracting the two funnels and covering their 3 feet diameter holes with water-tight plates, closing four mushroom-shaped air intake vents and about thirty other openings in the hull. These submarines had to be trimmed with great care. The large flat foredeck lacked buoyancy and produced a tendency to dive, as a result of which most of the class had at some time unintentionally nose-dived to the bottom. Occasionally, sea water entered through the air intakes and down the funnels, extinguishing the boiler fires, causing explosions, shorting out the electrical circuits and converting the boiler room into a flooded sauna.

In an attempt to correct some of the faults inherent in the original design, these submarines were all modified by lengthening the funnels and fitting bulbous *swan* bows, within which extra buoyancy tanks were installed. The forward gun was also removed as it proved impossible to man even in calm water at speeds over 12 knots.

K-13 sank on trials in the Gareloch in 1917 when she dived with the air intake vents still open. Of the 80 crew and dockyard men aboard, only 47 were saved after a rescue operation taking three days. She was raised and renumbered K-22.

THE EXERCISE. In a massive naval exercise, code named EC1, involving a large number of battleships and cruisers, 9 K-boats and numerous destroyers, two flotillas of Royal Navy ships left Rosyth after dark on the night of 31st January 1918, and steamed down the Forth at 19 knots in line astern, strung out over 20 miles, each following the shaded blue stern light of the vessel ahead. Radio silence was observed, and the navigation lights were switched off.

The first flotilla was led by the cruiser *Ithuriel*, followed by the K-11, K-17, K-14, K-12, and K-22, then the cruisers *Australia*, *New Zealand*, *Indomitable* and *Inflexible*. A few miles astern, the cruiser *Fearless* led the next flotilla consisting of the K-4, K-3, K-6 and K-7 followed by the battleships and destroyers.

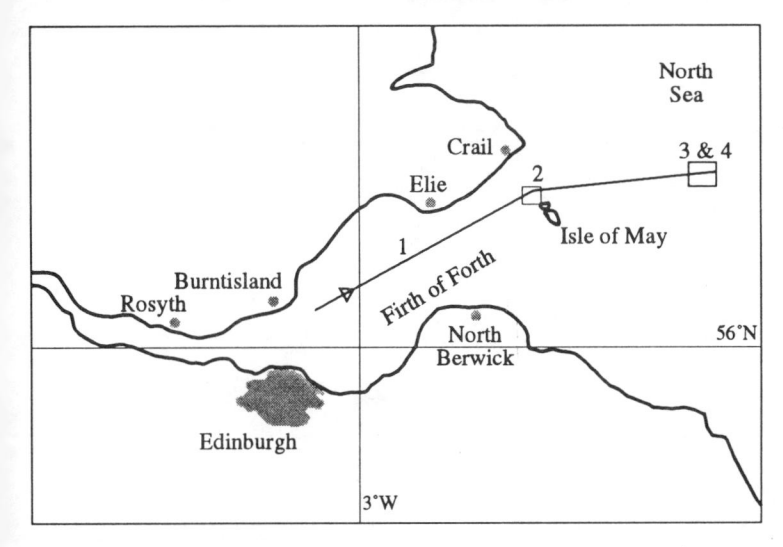

This diagram shows the scene of the Battle of May Island. The numbers refer to the various stages in the Battle shown in the diagram overleaf.

THE CAUSE. Ahead of them in the darkness and mist, a small group of mine sweepers was patrolling across their path, unaware of the fleet exercise in progress. On seeing them, K-11 reduced speed and turned to port, as did K-17. Approaching May Island, the commander of K-14 was suddenly aware that the K-17, (Lt. Cdr. H.J. Hearn), immediately ahead of him, had swerved to port, and at the same time saw two small vessels emerging from the mist to cross his bow. On taking avoiding action with full right rudder, the helm jammed in that position, causing the boat to continue in a circle clear of the K-12, but broadside into the path of the K-22 which was still running at 19 knots.

Unable to avoid her, the K-22 rammed into the K-14's port side, damaging her own bows, and slicing off the K-14's bows aft of the forward torpedo room. By closing watertight doors, immediate disaster was averted, but both submarines were now lying stopped in the water with flooded compartments in the path of the cruisers bearing down on them at 19 knots. Lights were switched on, flares fired and radio silence was broken as calls for assistance went out.

Three of the battle-cruisers swept past safely, their wash rolling the submarines violently, but the fourth, the *Inflexible*, smashed into the K-22, bending 30 feet of the submarine's already-damaged bows at right angles to the hull and shearing off a ballast tank as she rode over her, forcing the K-22 under the surface. As the cruiser continued on her way in the dark, apparently unaware that she had run down the submarine, the K-22 popped up again behind her and resumed calling for help.

THE ABORTIVE RESCUE. The *Ithuriel* picked up the distress calls from the submarines astern, but due to a decoding error, the erroneous impression gained in the *Ithuriel* was that a vessel named *Nova Scotia* had collided with the K-12! Twenty minutes later, the correct message was received, and *Ithuriel*, (by this time some 18 miles East of the May), turned back with

1. Ships involved in Exercise EC1, which resulted in the *Battle of May Island*

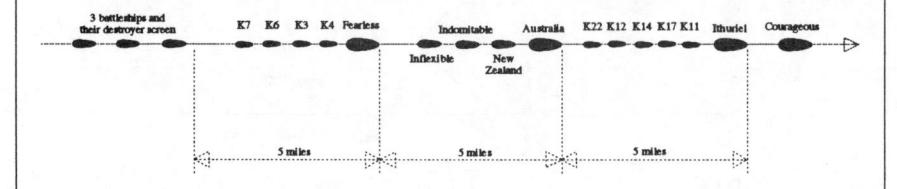

3 battleships and their destroyer screen — K7 K6 K3 K4 Fearless — Indomitable, Inflexible — Australia, New Zealand — K22 K12 K14 K17 K11 Ithuriel — Courageous

5 miles — 5 miles — 5 miles

2. The original collision between *K14* and *K22* at 7.15 pm

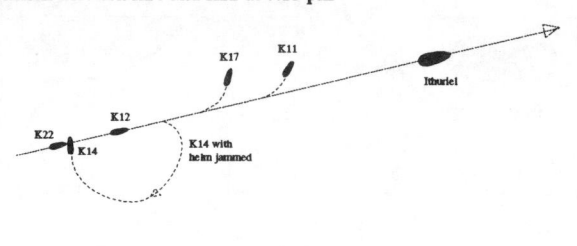

K17, K11, Ithuriel
K22, K12, K14 with helm jammed

May Island

26 minutes later, at 7.41 pm, the *Inflexible* struck the *K22*

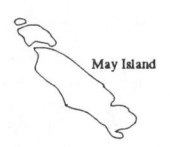

3. Turnback of *Ithuriel* and her submarines, and the collision between *Fearless* and *K17*

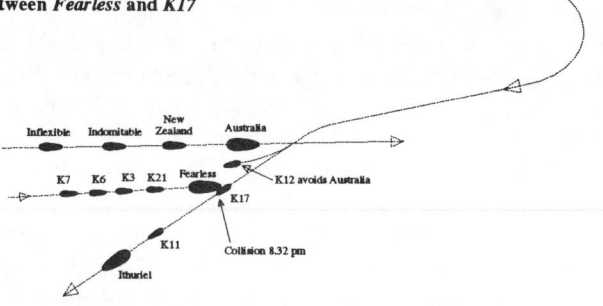

K12 K17 K11 Ithuriel

Inflexible, Indomitable, New Zealand, Australia
K7 K6 K3 K21 Fearless — K12 avoids Australia
K17
K11
Collision 8.32 pm
Ithuriel

4. The collision between *Fearless* and *K17*, then the collision between *K6* and *K4*

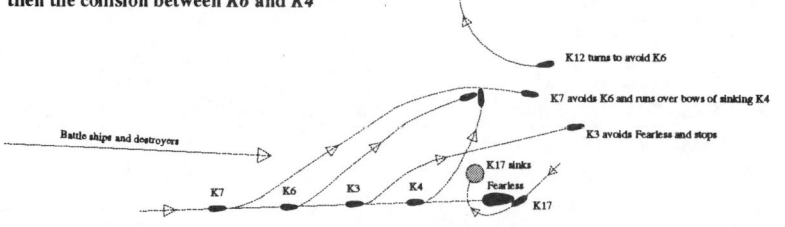

K12 turns to avoid K6
K7 avoids K6 and runs over bows of sinking K4
Battle ships and destroyers
K3 avoids Fearless and stops
K17 sinks
K7 K6 K3 K4 Fearless
K17

her remaining submarines to assist. Realising the danger of running headlong into the second flotilla of warships still steaming down river towards them, the navigation lights were turned on, but no radio message was sent out to warn the oncoming ships that she had turned back. *K-12* suddenly found the cruiser *Australia* bearing down on her. By luck they just missed each other, but were so close that the officers on *Australia* were able to look down the *K-12*'s funnels and see the glow of her furnaces!

The *Fearless*, leading the second wave of ships, had also picked up the distress calls and had switched her navigation lights on. At 7.54 pm she passed clear to the East of the May Island. According to the radio reports of the original collision, the danger area, a mile and a half North of the May, should have been safely astern, and speed was increased to 21 knots. Unfortunately, her commander was unaware that the *Ithuriel* and her submarines had turned back towards them, and very shortly both groups of ships met head on in the darkness and mists, thirteen miles East of the May Island.

THE FATAL CIRCUMSTANCES. At 8.32 pm the *Fearless* rammed into the *K-17* just forward of her conning tower, but all 56 crew managed to escape from the submarine in the eight minutes before she went down. The group swimming in the water stayed together, imagining that with the number of ships in the area, they would soon be picked up. Immediately behind the *Fearless*, the *K-4*, (Lt. Cdr. David de B. Stocks), turned to port and stopped. The *K-3* behind her did likewise, but overshot the *K-4*, closely scraping past to stop some distance away. The *K-6* then met the *K-12* coming back upriver on a collision course straight towards her, having only just narrowly avoided colliding with the *Australia*, and in taking avoiding action, the *K-6* rammed the *K-4*, almost slicing her in half. Entangled with each other, both submarines began to sink, and it was only by going full astern that the *K-6* managed to break free from the *K-4* to avoid being dragged to the bottom with her.

Seconds after the *K-4* turned over and sank, the *K-7* passed overhead, gently brushing her keel, and stopped to look for survivors. Her deck party were stripped off, ready to enter the water to help their fellow submariners, but there were no survivors from the *K-4*. Another of the shortcomings of the K-boats was that they were not equipped with any form of underwater escape apparatus.

THE FINAL DÉBACLE. By this time the battleships and destroyers following behind *Fearless* and her submarines arrived on the scene at 21 knots, and ploughed on through the cluster of damaged and confused ships, two of them missing the *K-3* by the thickness of her hull plating, and washing the *K-7*'s deck party off the casing, so that they too had to be rescued. In seconds, they passed the spot where the *K-17* had gone down, chopping up or sucking under and drowning the men still swimming in the water. By the time they passed by, only nine remained alive, one of whom died shortly after being picked up by the *K-7*.

News of this disastrous episode was suppressed at the time. It had cost almost 100 lives, the loss of two submarines, damage to three others and two surface ships, and later became known as the *Battle of May Island*.

CHAPTER 7

THE WRECKS OF FIFE NESS

INTRODUCTION

Fife Ness is the easternmost point of the ancient Kingdom of Fife. The sandy beach, flanked by rocks, shelves steeply and is dangerous for bathers. For other reasons, the headland and its shallow offling rocky islets and shoals is dangerous to shipping - witness the rash of ship wrecks just offshore.

For many years the North Carr lightship was the guardian of the North Carr Rock off Fife Ness. It has now been replaced by a beacon on the North Carr Rock and the old lightship is now preserved as a museum in Anstruther harbour.

The shore-based Fife Ness light is the location of HM Coastguard HQ for the Berwick to Montrose area. It is always worth phoning for the latest weather and sea conditions, and this is always helpful to a visiting diving party.

The entire coast is rocky, with off-lying reefs around Fife Ness, giving way to the sandy shores of St. Andrews Bay.

St. Monance is a busy fishing village on this popular and scenic section of the Fife coast Although it has a harbour, it has no slipway.

Pittenweem offers a sheltered harbour for the local fishing fleet but unfortunately has no slipway for use by visiting diving parties.

Anstruther harbour has the only launching site for this area at the lifeboat slip; this is more fully described in Chapter 6. Several of the fishing vessels which operate out of Anstruther are available for hire by diving parties. The local museum - the Scottish Fisheries Museum - provides a wealth of detail about past fishing activities along the East coast of Scotland.

Cellardyke, which provided the main harbour for Anstruther, was the principal port in Fife. Indeed, it was one of the main ports in the East of Scotland, having had a fleet of 221 boats in 1881 and employing nearly 600 fishermen. The long decline to the present state of Scotland's fishing industry is well known.

The tiny, quaint harbour at the fishing village of Crail is home to local crab and lobster boats, but again there is no slipway.

— Fife Ness —

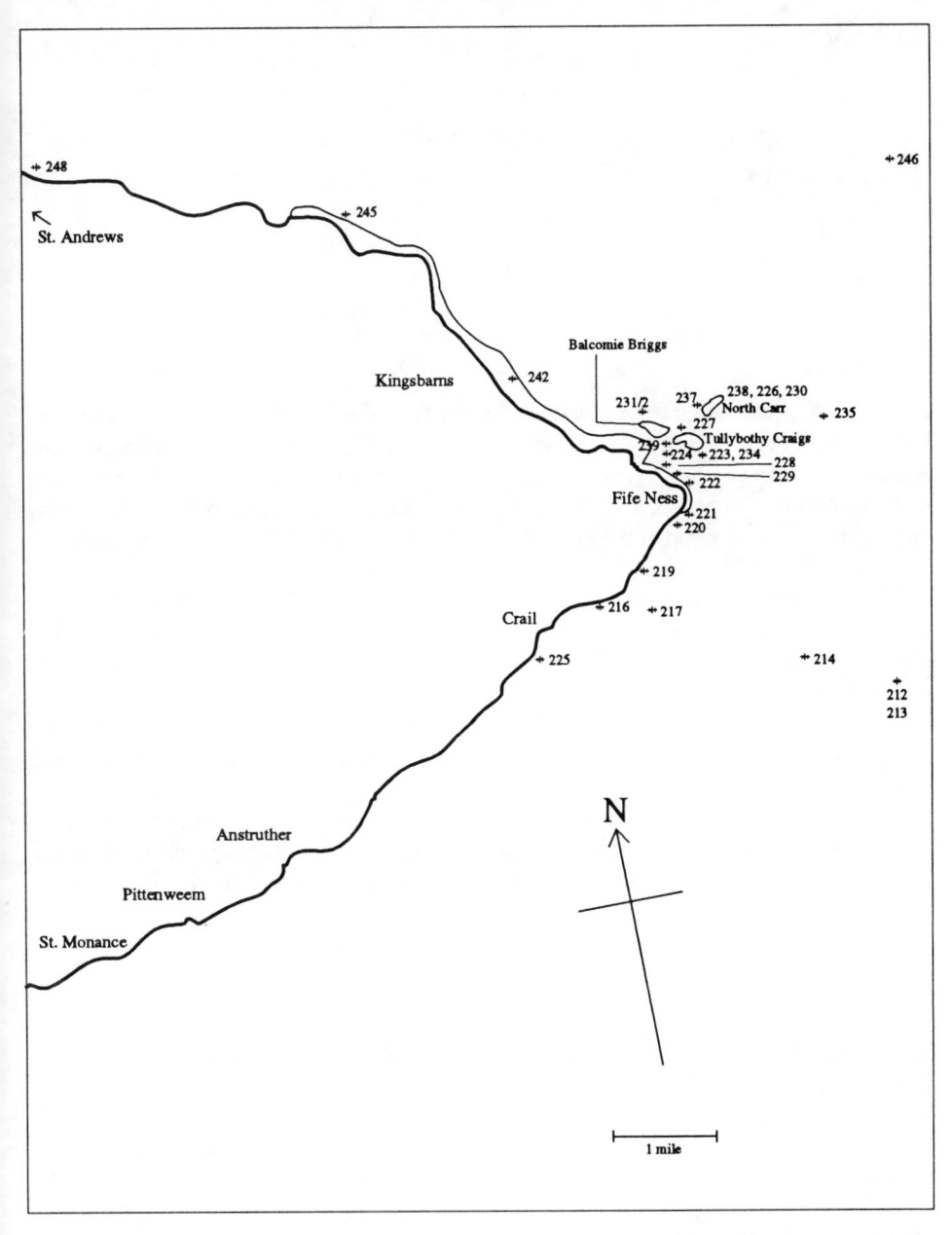

Chart of the wrecks around the Fife Ness area. Note the clustering of shipping losses at Fife Ness and its offlying shoals.

THE WRECKS

LEONARD

Wreck No :	210	Date Sunk :	12 02 1920
Latitude :		Longitude :	
Decca Lat :		Decca Long :	
Location :	Lost Inverkeithing to Dundee	Area :	Fife Ness
Type :	Drifter	Tonnage :	
Length : feet Beam : feet		Draught :	feet
How Sunk :		Depth :	metres

HM drifter *Leonard* sailed from Inverkeithing on Thursday 12th February 1920, bound for Dundee, but never arrived, and was lost with all hands. The crew of nine according to some accounts, and six according to others, had been employed for some time in delivering vessels to be reconditioned by the Admiralty, from port to port. Vessels surplus to Admiralty requirements after the end of the First World War, (and, indeed, the Second World War), were reconditioned before being returned to civilian use.

She could be somewhere in the Forth, or off Fife Ness, or perhaps on the sand banks off the mouth of the Tay. Statistically, it is most likely that she ran aground in the Forth, but if that was the case, one might perhaps have expected either wreckage or bodies to have been found washed ashore somewhere.

If she had been involved in a collision with another vessel, the colliding vessel would surely have reported the matter, particularly if she herself had been damaged, as the owner would no doubt have sought an explanation.

The third possibility is that she may have simply foundered, any flotsam being swept out to sea unseen. In that case, she may be one of the many *Unknowns* waiting to be investigated.

My personal guess is that she may have become another victim of the North Carr Rock.

STORJEN (OB 71)

Wreck No :	211	Date Sunk :	02 07 1978
Latitude :	56 14 51 N	Longitude :	02 27 12 W
Decca Lat :	5614.80 N	Decca Long :	0227.20 W
Location :	5 miles ESE of Fife Ness	Area :	Fife Ness
Type :	MFV	Tonnge :	
Length : feet Beam : feet		Draught :	feet
How Sunk : Fire		Depth :	51 metres

Storjen sank after a fire. Charted as a wreck with at least 40 metres over it in 51 metres.

OTHONNA

Wreck No :	212	Date Sunk :	20 04 1917
Latitude :	56 15 00 N PA	Longitude :	02 30 00 W PA
Decca Lat :	5615.00 N	Decca Long :	0230.00 W
Location :	Off Fife Ness	Area :	Fife Ness
Type :	Trawler	Tonnage :	180 gross
Length :	110.8 feet Beam : 20.8 feet	Draught :	11.1 feet
How Sunk :	Mined	Depth :	36 metres

The *Othonna* was a steel screw ketch, (steam trawler), built in 1899 by J. Duthie & Son, Aberdeen, engine by Whyte & Mair, Dundee.

She was sunk by a mine on 20th April 1917. The approximate position 561500N, 023000W dates from 24/3/1919.

The depth at this position is 36 metres, but varies from 30 to 50 metres within a radius of 1 mile. Asdic searches in this position in 1955, 1960, 1977 failed to find any trace.

Another, apparently more accurate position very close by at 561455N, 022950W, also dates from 1919. These positions are so close to each other (only 800 feet apart), that it seems unlikely that an asdic search around the first position would fail to detect a wreck in the second position.

SPEY

Wreck No :	213	Date Sunk :	
Latitude :	56 15 00 N PA	Longitude :	02 30 00 W PA
Decca Lat :	5615.00 N	Decca Long :	0230.00 W
Location :	Off Fife Ness ?	Area :	Fife Ness
Type :	Steamship	Tonnage :	659 gross
Length :	feet Beam : feet	Draught :	feet
How Sunk :		Depth :	metres

The 659 ton steamship *Spey* was reported as having sunk "off Fife". The approximate Lat/Long has been derived from the supposition that the *Spey* sank off Fife Ness.

LINGBANK

Wreck No :	214	Date Sunk :	26 04 1927
Latitude :	56 15 10 N PA	Longitude :	02 32 50 W PA
Decca Lat :	5615.17 N	Decca Long :	0232.83 W
Location :	Off Fife Ness	Area :	Fife Ness
Type :	Trawler	Tonnage :	257 gross

Length :	132.0 feet	Beam : 22.0 feet	Draught : 10.8 feet
How Sunk :	Foundered		Depth : 17 metres

Lingbank was a German steam trawler sunk 26/4/1927. In 1927 the position was given as 561510N, 023250W, 2 miles 141.5° from Fife Ness, and charted as Wk PA, but was not located by *HMS Scott* in 1960.

UNKNOWN

Wreck No :	215	Date Sunk :	
Latitude :	56 15 27 N	Longitude :	02 22 54 W
Decca Lat :	5615.45 N	Decca Long :	0222.90 W
Location :	7 miles ESE of Fife Ness	Area :	Fife Ness
Type :		Tonnage :	
Length : feet	Beam : feet	Draught :	feet
How Sunk :		Depth :	51 metres

This wreck is in two parts, which might provide a clue to the reason for her sinking - possibly mined or torpedoed? Could she be the *Spey* or the *Othonna*?

SAVANT

Wreck No :	216	Date Sunk :	07 02 1883
Latitude :	56 15 30 N PA	Longitude :	02 36 00 W PA
Decca Lat :	5615.50 N	Decca Long :	0236.00 W
Location :	1/4 mile E. of Crail Harbour	Area :	Fife Ness
Type :	Schooner	Tonnage :	106 gross
Length :	81.6 feet Beam : 22.2 feet	Draught :	10.7 feet
How Sunk :	Ran aground	Depth :	3 metres

The Welsh schooner *Savant*, en route from Middlesbrough to Swansea with a cargo of pig iron, encountered a severe SSE storm, Force 10, and was blown North before it, finally being dashed ashore 1/4 mile East of Crail harbour on 7th February 1883. Three of the crew were rescued by rocket apparatus, but the captain and a boy were drowned.

RIVER AVON

Wreck No :	217	Date Sunk :	07 02 1937
Latitude :	56 15 38 N	Longitude :	02 35 30 W

―――――――― Fife Ness ――――――――

Decca Lat :	5615.63 N	Decca Long :	0235.50 W
Location :	Kilminning Rock, Fife Ness	Area :	Fife Ness
Type :	Trawler	Tonnage :	202 gross
Length :	115.4 feet Beam : 22.5 feet	Draught :	12.1 feet
How Sunk :	Ran aground	Depth :	5 metres

The Granton-registered steam trawler *River Avon* ran on to Kilminning Rock, about ³/₄ mile South West of Fife Ness, at 11.30 pm on 7th February 1937.

She was of steel construction, built by Rennie, Forrest of Wivenhoe in 1919.

PLADDA

Wreck No :	218	Date Sunk :	14 12 1890
Latitude :	56 15 45 N	Longitude :	02 36 00 W
Decca Lat :	5615.75 N	Decca Long :	0236.00 W
Location :	Ashore on rocks 1 mile E of Crail	Area :	Fife Ness
Type :	Steamship	Tonnage :	421 gross
Length :	181.5 feet Beam : 23.1 feet	Draught :	13.2 feet
How Sunk :	Ran aground	Depth :	5 metres

The Dundee iron steamship *Pladda*, 239 tons net, went ashore on rocks about 1 mile East of Crail while en route from Newcastle to Dundee on 14th December 1890.

CHINGFORD

Wreck No :	219	Date Sunk :	23 12 1924
Latitude :	56 15 58 N	Longitude :	02 35 46 W
Decca Lat :	5615.97 N	Decca Long :	0235.77 W
Location :	Sauchope, near Crail	Area :	Fife Ness
Type :	Steamship	Tonnage :	1517 gross
Length :	264.5 feet Beam : 37.0 feet	Draught :	17.8 feet
How Sunk :	Ran aground	Depth :	6 metres

The Dundee steamship *Chingford*, built in 1889, was driven ashore on Kilminning Sands, Crail, during a severe South Westerly storm. She had been en route from Transgund and Dundee to Grangemouth with a cargo of timber.

Anstruther and Brought Ferry lifeboats went to her assistance, but when they arrived, great rollers were sweeping over the vessel and sending up huge clouds of spray. Crail LSA rushed to the scene and made efforts to get a line to the stricken ship, to rescue captain Chapman and his crew of 20.

The keel, propeller shaft and 4-bladed propeller with squared-off blade ends lie close to the shore off the caravan site at Crail. The forward end of the keel is just visible above water at low tide.

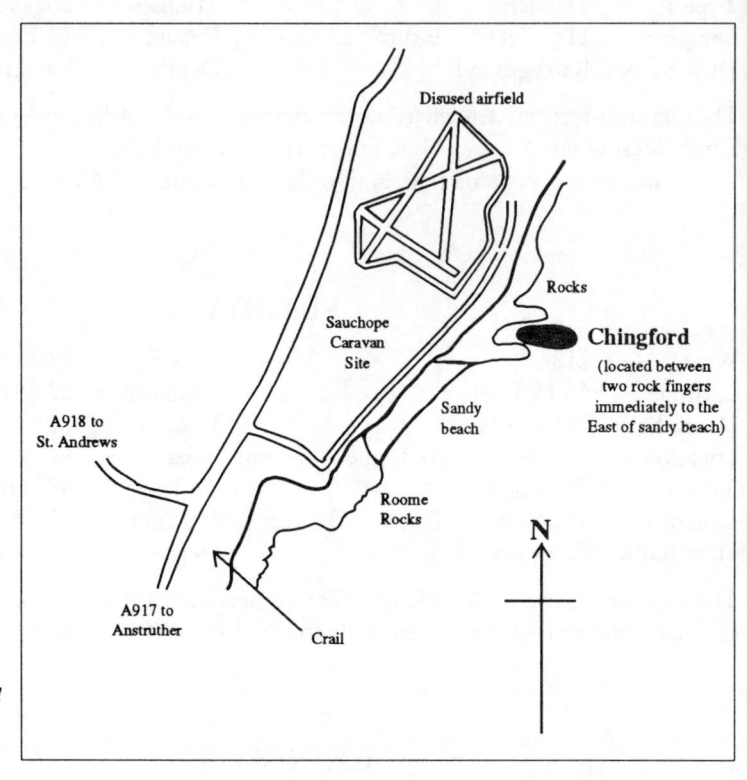

The Chingford, wrecked off the beach off Sauchope Caravan Site

LOUISE

Wreck No :	220	**Date Sunk :**	23 10 1881
Latitude :	56 16 00 N PA	**Longitude :**	02 33 00 W PA
Decca Lat :	5616.00 N	**Decca Long :**	0233.00 W
Location :	1 mile E of Crail	**Area :**	Fife Ness
Type :	Schooner	**Tonnage :**	260 gross
Length :	feet **Beam :** feet	**Draught :**	feet
How Sunk :	Ran aground	**Depth :**	10 metres

The Norwegian schooner *Louise*, from Tonsberg to Newcastle with a cargo of pit props, was blown ashore one mile East of Crail by a Force 9 severe gale from the East South East on 23rd October 1881. She was 147 tons net.

JANE ROSS

Wreck No :	221	Date Sunk :	14 09 1934
Latitude :	56 16 08 N	Longitude :	02 35 36 W
Decca Lat :	5616.13 N	Decca Long :	0235.60 W
Location :	Kilminning Point	Area :	Fife Ness
Type :	Trawler	Tonnage :	184 gross
Length :	110.1 feet Beam : 21.2 feet	Draught :	11.6 feet
How Sunk :	Ran aground	Depth :	metres

The Aberdeen steam trawler *Jane Ross*, built in 1901 by Hall & Co. of Aberdeen, was making for Methil to replenish her coal bunkers when she ran aground in thick fog at Kilminning Point, two miles from Crail. The Crail fishing boat *Maypole* managed to get alongside the *Jane Ross* and took off the nine crew who were landed safely at Crail.

VILDFUGL

Wreck No :	222	Date Sunk :	28 05 1951
Latitude :	56 16 45 N	Longitude :	02 35 00 W
Decca Lat :	5616.75 N	Decca Long :	0235.00 W
Location :	Ashore at Fife Ness	Area :	Fife Ness
Type :	Tanker	Tonnage :	477 gross
Length :	156.1 feet Beam : 25.6 feet	Draught :	10.9 feet
How Sunk :	Ran aground	Depth :	12 metres

The small Norwegian tanker *Vildfugl*, built in 1941, ran ashore at 1.55 am on Fife Ness Point while en route in ballast, from Inverness to Grangemouth. She broke into three parts, and became a total loss.

DOWNIEHILLS

Wreck No :	223	Date Sunk :	18 01 1926
Latitude :	56 16 46 N PA	Longitude :	02 34 52 W PA
Decca Lat :	5616.77 N	Decca Long :	0234.87 W
Location :	PA 1/4 mile NE of Fife Ness	Area :	Fife Ness
Type :	Trawler	Tonnage :	227 gross
Length :	117.1 feet Beam : 22.1 feet	Draught :	12.6 feet
How Sunk :	Ran aground	Depth :	10 metres

En route from Aberdeen to Methil, the Peterhead steam trawler *Downiehills* stranded at Fife Ness during the night, having failed to see the North Carr lightship in thick fog.

In a thrilling rescue which took only ten minutes, but which was witnessed by a crowd of over three hundred, the skipper and crew of four were rescued by the Crail life-saving apparatus which had to be brought three miles to the scene. Five minutes after the rocket line was shot across the ship, which lay 300 yards out, the first man was hauled safely ashore. *Downiehills* was a steel screw ketch built in 1917 by Hawthorns of Leith.

ANDREAS

Wreck No :	224	Date Sunk :	16 12 1879
Latitude :	56 17 00 N PA	Longitude :	02 35 00 W PA
Decca Lat :	5617.00 N	Decca Long :	0235.00 W
Location :	Fife Ness	Area :	Fife Ness
Type :	Brig	Tonnage :	192 gross
Length :	feet Beam : feet	Draught :	feet
How Sunk :	Ran aground	Depth :	10 metres

The Norwegian brig *Andreas*, from Marans, France to Leith with a cargo of beans was lost on Fife Ness on 16th December 1879.

QUEEN

Wreck No :	225	Date Sunk :	18 04 1857
Latitude :	56 17 00 N	Longitude :	02 34 30 W
Decca Lat :	5617.00 N	Decca Long :	0234.50 W
Location :	Carr Rocks off Fife Ness	Area :	Fife Ness
Type :	Paddle steamer	Tonnage :	602 gross
Length :	183.0 feet Beam : 26.0 feet	Draught :	14.5 feet
How Sunk :	Ran aground	Depth :	12 metres

The iron paddle steamer *Queen*, built in 1845, was wrecked on Carr Rocks off Fife Ness. She was later beached at Crail, but broke up in storms on 25/4/1857 at 561500N, 023730W.

KNOT

Wreck No :	226	Date Sunk :	05 11 1916
Latitude :	56 17 00 N	Longitude :	02 34 30 W
Decca Lat :	5617.00 N	Decca Long :	0234.50 W
Location :	On North Carr Rock, Fife Ness	Area :	Fife Ness
Type :	Trawler	Tonnage :	168 gross
Length :	110.3 feet Beam : 20.9 feet	Draught :	11.1 feet
How Sunk :	Ran aground	Depth :	12 metres

The position given was reported on 24/3/1919, but no wreck was located here by HMS *Scott* in 1959. This is hardly surprising, as it will be well broken up and scattered, making it impossible to distinguish from the rocky bottom by echo sounder or A/S.

Knot was a steel screw ketch (steam trawler) built in 1903 by Goole S.B. & Rprg. Co., and engined by C.D. Holmes of Hull.

COMMODORE

Wreck No :	227	Date Sunk :	16 09 1859
Latitude :	56 17 00 N PA	Longitude :	02 35 00 W PA
Decca Lat :	5617.00 N	Decca Long :	0235.00 W
Location :	Fife Ness	Area :	Fife Ness
Type :	Paddle steamer	Tonnage :	705 gross
Length :	172.6 feet Beam : 24.3 feet	Draught :	7.5 feet
How Sunk :	Ran aground	Depth :	metres

This *Commodore* was a wooden paddle steamer built in 1837 for service on the West coast of Scotland, but was soon transferred to the Liverpool-Southampton-Le Havre route in connection with Cunard. She was later sold in 1855 to the Aberdeen Steam Navigation Co., and was wrecked on Fife Ness on 16/9/1859.

She is not to be confused with another *Commodore* which was an iron paddle steamer built in 1875 as the *Flying Meteor* by J.T. Eltringham, engine by J.P. Rennoldson. She was renamed *Gladstone* in 1882, and finally renamed *Commodore* in 1890. She was stranded and wrecked at St. Andrews on 11/12/1896. (See *Gladstone*).

ANNETTE

Wreck No :	228	Date Sunk :	14 07 1879
Latitude :	56 17 00 N PA	Longitude :	02 35 00 W PA
Decca Lat :	5617.00 N	Decca Long :	0235.00 W
Location :	Fife Ness	Area :	Fife Ness
Type :	Brig	Tonnage :	164 gross
Length :	feet Beam : feet	Draught :	feet
How Sunk :	Ran aground	Depth :	10 metres

The Norwegian brig *Annette*, from Christiania (Oslo), to Leith with a cargo of pit props was blown ashore on Fife Ness in a severe North Easterly gale, Force 9, on 14th July 1879.

JUNO

Wreck No :	229	Date Sunk :	09 04 1879
Latitude :	56 17 00 N PA	Longitude :	02 35 00 W PA
Decca Lat :	5617.00 N	Decca Long :	0235.00 W
Location :	Near N. Carr Beacon	Area :	Fife Ness
Type :	Schooner	Tonnage :	104 gross
Length :	feet Beam : feet	Draught :	feet
How Sunk :	Ran aground	Depth :	10 metres

The German schooner *Juno*, en route from Delfzyl, Holland, to Grangemouth with a cargo of straw was stranded and beached at the North Carr beacon. Wind at the time was Force 6 from the East South East.

FAIRY QUEEN

Wreck No :	230	Date Sunk :	28 12 1877
Latitude :	56 17 12 N	Longitude :	02 34 30 W
Decca Lat :	5617.20 N	Decca Long :	0234.50 W
Location :	Balcomie Briggs, Fife Ness	Area :	Fife Ness
Type :	Steamship	Tonnage :	229 gross
Length :	feet Beam : feet	Draught :	feet
How Sunk :	Ran aground	Depth :	8 metres

The 229 ton iron steamship *Fairy Queen* was en route from Stromness to Leith in ballast when she struck North Carr rocks in a Force 6 S by W wind on 28th December 1877.

BJORNHAUG

Wreck No :	231	Date Sunk :	05 04 1940
Latitude :	56 17 12 N	Longitude :	02 34 30 W
Decca Lat :	5617.20 N	Decca Long :	0234.50 W
Location :	Balcomie Briggs, Fife Ness	Area :	Fife Ness
Type :	Steamship	Tonnage :	443 gross
Length :	feet Beam : feet	Draught :	feet
How Sunk :	Ran aground	Depth :	8 metres

The 443 ton steamship *Bjornhaug* ran ashore on Balcomie Briggs near Fife Ness while en route from Copenhagen to London with a cargo of paper on 5th April 1940.

The wreck is broken up and scattered, making it impossible to distinguish from the rocky bottom by echo sounder.

MUSKETEER

Wreck No : 232
Latitude : 56 17 12 N
Decca Lat : 5617.20 N
Location : Balcomie Briggs, Fife Ness
Type : Trawler
Length :   feet   Beam :   feet
How Sunk : Ran aground

Date Sunk :
Longitude : 02 34 30 W
Decca Long : 0234.50 W
Area : Fife Ness
Tonnage : 384 gross
Draught :   feet
Depth : 10 metres

Musketeer was an armed trawler. The date of her loss is unknown, but was presumably during the First World War.

EINAR JARL

Wreck No : 233
Latitude : 56 17 30 N PA
Decca Lat : 5617.50 N
Location : 9.75 miles E of Fife Ness
Type : Steamship
Length : 265.3 feet   Beam : 42.1 feet
How Sunk : Mined

Date Sunk : 17 03 1941
Longitude : 02 18 00 W PA
Decca Long : 0218.00 W
Area : Fife Ness
Tonnage : 1858 gross
Draught : 17.9 feet
Depth : 53 metres

Einar Jarl was a Norwegian steamship mined en route from Hull to Halifax, Nova Scotia in ballast. She was built in 1921, had one deck, and was registered in Trondheim. One member of the crew of 21 (a Greek), was lost.

Lloyds gave the position as 561730N, 021800W, hence the wreck charted as PA in this position. The Norwegian Maritime Directorate gives 561800N, 021800W PA. The nearest accurately charted wreck is at 561736N, 021930W, but this is reported to be only 40 metres long (132 feet). The next nearest charted wreck is at 561858N, 021712W, and this wreck is reported to be 95 metres long (313.5 feet).

Neither of these matches the 265 feet (80 metres) length of the *Einar Jarl*.

WINDSOR CASTLE

Wreck No : 234
Latitude : 56 17 30 N PA
Decca Lat : 5617.50 N
Location : 2 miles E of Crail

Date Sunk : 01 10 1844
Longitude : 02 35 00 W PA
Decca Long : 0235.00 W
Area : Fife Ness

Type :	Paddle steamer		Tonnage :	151 gross
Length :	130.0 feet	Beam : 18.5 feet	Draught :	feet
How Sunk :	Ran aground		Depth :	12 metres

The iron paddle steamer *Windsor Castle* was built in 1838 by Tod & McGregor, Glasgow.

She collided with Carr beacon off Fife Ness while en route from the Tay to Leith. For a short time her course was maintained, but finding that his vessel was sinking, the master turned towards land and grounded her with her boiler room flooded, two miles East of Crail. (This puts her very close to Fife Ness).

Windsor Castle had only one boat, capable of holding six persons, and one oar, but three fishing boats assisted with the rescue of those on board. Holes made in the hull by the anchor being driven in were patched up, but when the tide came in the vessel rolled on to the rocks where she broke up.

ISLANDMAGEE

Wreck No :	235		Date Sunk :	26 10 1953
Latitude :	56 17 30 N		Longitude :	02 32 18 W
Decca Lat :	5617.50 N		Decca Long :	0232.30 W
Location :	Off Fife Ness		Area :	Fife Ness
Type :	Steamship		Tonnage :	227 gross
Length :	117.0 feet	Beam : 22.0 feet	Draught :	10.0 feet
How Sunk :	Foundered		Depth :	29 metres

The *Islandmagee* sank during a Force 9 severe gale. Six of the crew were lost, as were six of the crew of the Arbroath lifeboat *Robert Lindsay* which was attempting to assist.

The wreck was positively identified as the *Islandmagee* by the builders plate and bell which were recovered in 1986.

The wreck is intact, standing 6 metres high. Depth to the top of the wreck is 34 metres and, to the seabed of rock and sand, 40 metres. There is one forward hold and the engine is aft. A large grab lies on the starboard side of the wreck.

The 1990 chart shows the wreck at 561745N 023224W, but the correct position is 561730N 023218W.

UNKNOWN

Wreck No :	236	Date Sunk :	
Latitude :	56 17 36 N	Longitude :	02 19 30 W
Decca Lat :	5617.55 N	Decca Long :	0219.50 W
Location :	8.5 miles E of Fife Ness	Area :	Fife Ness

―――――― Fife Ness ――――――

Type :				Tonnage :	
Length :	132.0 feet	Beam :	feet	Draught :	feet
How Sunk :				Depth :	47 metres

The wreck charted at 561736N, 021930W is reported to be 40 metres long (132 feet). Could this be the *Bodo*? (139 feet long).

The *Lingbank*, for which an accurate position is unknown, was 132 feet long.

MARIE ELIZABETH

Wreck No :	237			Date Sunk :	26 11 1885
Latitude :	56 17 36 N PA			Longitude :	02 34 30 W PA
Decca Lat :	5617.60 N			Decca Long :	0234.50 W
Location :	W side of Carr Rocks			Area :	Fife Ness
Type :	Schooner			Tonnage :	209 gross
Length :	feet	Beam :	feet	Draught :	feet
How Sunk :	Ran aground			Depth :	metres

The Russian schooner *Marie Elizabeth* was driven ashore on the West side of Carr Rocks, about 1 mile North East of Fife Ness, on 26th November 1885 while en route from Folkestone to South Shields in ballast. The vessel was observed ashore at daybreak, and Crail rocket apparatus was sent to the spot. Although a line was successfully fired aboard the vessel, the crew failed to take advantage of it. Two of them were washed ashore and rescued, but the remaining five were drowned.

OLIVIER

Wreck No :	238			Date Sunk :	07 03 1881
Latitude :	56 17 36 N			Longitude :	02 34 30 W
Decca Lat :	5617.60 N			Decca Long :	0234.50 W
Location :	Carr Rock, Fife Ness			Area :	Fife Ness
Type :	Brig			Tonnage :	266 gross
Length :	feet	Beam :	feet	Draught :	feet
How Sunk :	Ran aground			Depth :	12 metres

The Norwegian brig *Olivier*, en route from Ymuiden to Newcastle in ballast, ran on to Carr Rock, Fife Ness in calm conditions on 7th March 1881. She was obviously well off course!

FESTING GRINDALL

Wreck No :	239	Date Sunk :	04 10 1928
Latitude :	56 17 45 N	Longitude :	02 34 30 W
Decca Lat :	5617.75 N	Decca Long :	0234.50 W
Location :	Ashore 1 mile N of Fife Ness	Area :	Fife Ness
Type :	Trawler	Tonnage :	236 gross
Length :	117.0 feet Beam : 23.0 feet	Draught :	13.0 feet
How Sunk :	Ran aground	Depth :	10 metres

Festing Grindall was a steam trawler built in 1917 by Smiths Dock at Middlesbrough. She ran ashore in fog 1 mile North (True) from Fife Ness Point on a voyage from Aberdeen to Granton for coal. The crew of nine landed in their own boat. The vessel was very badly damaged and became a total wreck. The position given above is not immediately adjacent to the shore, but on the outlying Tullybothy Craigs, which uncover at low water.

UNKNOWN

Wreck No :	240	Date Sunk :	
Latitude :	56 17 48 N	Longitude :	02 24 06 W
Decca Lat :	5617.80 N	Decca Long :	0224.10 W
Location :	6 miles E of Fife Ness	Area :	Fife Ness
Type :		Tonnage :	
Length :	100.0 feet Beam : feet	Draught :	feet
How Sunk :		Depth :	45 metres

The wreck charted 6 miles East of Fife Ness is apparently 100 feet long.

KATE THOMPSON

Wreck No :	241	Date Sunk :	09 01 1895
Latitude :	56 17 50 N	Longitude :	02 37 24 W
Decca Lat :	5617.83 N	Decca Long :	0237.40 W
Location :	On rocks $2^{1}/_{4}$ miles N of Crail (PA)	Area :	Fife Ness
Type :	Steamship	Tonnage :	259 gross
Length :	feet Beam : feet	Draught :	feet
How Sunk :	Ran aground	Depth :	5 metres

The Newcastle-registered steel steamship *Kate Thompson* became a total loss after stranding on rocks 2 $^{1}/_{4}$ miles North of Crail, or 2 miles East of Anstruther, while en route from Dundee to Leith in ballast on 9th January 1895. She was 154 tons net.

— Fife Ness —

SUCCESS

Wreck No :	242	Date Sunk :	27 12 1914
Latitude :	56 18 00 N	Longitude :	02 37 36 W
Decca Lat :	5618.00 N	Decca Long :	0237.60 W
Location :	Cambo Sands, Kingsbarns	Area :	Fife Ness
Type :	Destroyer	Tonnage :	385 gross
Length :	214.5 feet Beam : 21.0 feet	Draught :	10.8 feet
How Sunk :	Ran aground	Depth :	1 metres

HMS *Success* was a destroyer built in 1901 by W. Doxford & Sons.

Only the keel remains, buried in the sand. A notice on the beach at Kingsbarns, and a photograph hanging in the village hall are reminders of the wrecking of the ship.

HARLEY

Wreck No :	243	Date Sunk :	14 11 1944
Latitude :	56 18 54 N	Longitude :	02 09 12 W
Decca Lat :	5618.90 N	Decca Long :	0209.20 W
Location :	15 miles E of Fife Ness	Area :	Fife Ness
Type :	Steamship	Tonnage :	400 gross
Length :	133.3 feet Beam : 24.1 feet	Draught :	11.2 feet
How Sunk :	Foundered	Depth :	58 metres

The steamship *Harley* was built in 1919 by A. De Jong.

While off Fife Ness she was overwhelmed by stress of weather and foundered with the loss of seven of her crew.

Charted as a wreck with at least 27 metres over it in about 56 metres.

UNKNOWN - ROCKINGHAM ?

Wreck No :	244	Date Sunk :	
Latitude :	56 19 00 N	Longitude :	02 17 12 W
Decca Lat :	5619.00 N	Decca Long :	0217.20 W
Location :	10 miles E of Fife Ness	Area :	Fife Ness
Type :		Tonnage :	
Length :	313.5 feet Beam : feet	Draught :	feet
How Sunk :		Depth :	41 metres

The wreck charted at 561900N, 021712W, 10 miles East of Fife Ness is reported to be 95 metres long (313.5 feet), with a minimum depth of 41 metres in about 50 metres.

This is obviously a fairly substantial ship and as an aid to establishing her identity, it would be helpful to know when the wreck was first discovered.

It may be HMS *Rockingham* (ex-USS *Swasey*), one of fifty World War One 4-stack, flush-deck American destroyers acquired under the Lend-lease Act 1940. Built by Bethlehem SB Co. in 1919, she was 1190 tons displacement, measured 311.0 x 40.0 x 10.0 feet and was armed with four 4" guns and twelve torpedo tubes. According to *British Vessels Lost at Sea 1939-45* she was lost by striking a mine "off East Scotland" on 27 September 1944.

GLOAMIN

Wreck No :	245	Date Sunk :	24 01 1881
Latitude :	56 19 30 N PA	Longitude :	02 40 00 W PA
Decca Lat :	5619.50 N	Decca Long :	0240.00 W
Location :	Near Boarhills	Area :	Fife Ness
Type :	Steamship	Tonnage :	791 gross
Length :	201.8 feet Beam : 27.1 feet	Draught :	14.5 feet
How Sunk :	Ran aground	Depth :	metres

The 487 ton net iron screw steamship *Gloamin*, built by Thompson of Dundee in 1880, stranded near Boarhills on 24th January 1881.

BLACKWHALE

Wreck No :	246	Date Sunk :	31 01 1918
Latitude :	56 20 00 N PA	Longitude :	02 30 00 W PA
Decca Lat :	5620.00 N	Decca Long :	0230.00 W
Location :	Off Fife Ness	Area :	Fife Ness
Type :	Whaler	Tonnage :	237 gross
Length :	feet Beam : feet	Draught :	feet
How Sunk :	Mined	Depth :	metres

The 237 ton whaler *Blackwhale* was mined off Fife Ness on 31st January 1918.

SALEM

Wreck No :	247	Date Sunk :	03 11 1914
Latitude :	56 20 05 N	Longitude :	02 48 00 W
Decca Lat :	5620.42 N	Decca Long :	0248.00 W
Location :	N side of St. Andrews Bay	Area :	Fife Ness
Type :	Barque	Tonnage :	438 gross

Length :	128.1 feet Beam : 29.2 feet	Draught :	17.1 feet
How Sunk :	Ran aground	Depth :	metres

The 438 ton Norwegian wooden barque *Salem* built in 1873, ran aground at the North end of St. Andrews Bay on 3rd November 1914.

GLADSTONE

Wreck No :	248	Date Sunk :	11 12 1896
Latitude :	56 20 30 N PA	Longitude :	02 47 00 W PA
Decca Lat :	5620.50 N	Decca Long :	0247.00 W
Location :	At St. Andrews	Area :	Fife Ness
Type :	Paddle steamer	Tonnage :	157 gross
Length :	118.0 feet Beam : 19.8 feet	Draught :	10.4 feet
How Sunk :	Ran aground	Depth :	metres

The iron paddle steamer *Flying Meteor*, built in 1875 by J.T. Eltringham, engine by J.P. Rennoldson, was renamed *Gladstone* in 1882. She was finally renamed *Commodore* in 1890, and was stranded and wrecked at St. Andrews on 11th December 1896.

Another *Gladstone*, a steam barque (was there really such a type of vessel?), of 20 tons net was stranded at the entrance to Granton on 9/11/1898.

MERLIN

Wreck No :	249	Date Sunk :	05 03 1881
Latitude :	56 20 30 N	Longitude :	02 47 15 W
Decca Lat :	5620.50 N	Decca Long :	0247.25 W
Location :	Old Castle, St. Andrews	Area :	Fife Ness
Type :	Barque	Tonnage :	367 gross
Length :	121.8 feet Beam : 27.5 feet	Draught :	17.1 feet
How Sunk :	Ran aground	Depth :	metres

The 367 ton barque *Merlin* was lost when she ran aground near the Old Castle at St. Andrews on 5th March 1881.

The vessel was built by Potts of Sunderland in 1865.

Chapter 8

The Wrecks of the Tay & Arbroath

Introduction

The coastline between Fife Ness and the River Tay is low-lying, and the mouth of the Tay is shallow, with a huge mass of moving sand stretching over 20 miles out to sea. In fact, this sand has almost covered some of the wrecks in St. Andrew's Bay

Northwards from the Tay, the coast from Arbroath to Lunan Bay is rocky with cliffs which are more than 200 feet high in places, and honeycombed with caves beloved of smugglers in bygone times.

The old and traditional university town of St. Andrews is the home of the game of golf and is also a picturesque fishing village with a small harbour.

Dundee, lying several miles upriver on the River Tay, is an important port with a long history. The centre of the world's jute trade in the 1830s, the port can now handle vessels up to oil tankers. Dundee was also the centre of a ship-building industry. Furthermore, quite a number of the vessels described in this book were Dundee-bound prior to their loss. Dundee was a wartime base for both submarines and destroyers.

Arbroath, where Robert the Bruce proclaimed Scotland's independence in 1320, is a fishing town famous for its *smokies* amongst other things.

Auchmithie, some two miles North east of Arbroath, is perched at the top of a 150 feet high cliff down which a steep track leads to the minute harbour and shingle beach. With difficulty (4 x 4 vehicles and a long length of rope) launching and recovery is possible across the stony beach at the foot of these cliffs.

Bell Rock (also known as Inchcape Rock) lies offshore some 10 miles SE of Arbroath, 11 miles NE of Fife Ness. This treacherous reef of red sandstone is reputed to have claimed countless ships before Robert Stevenson, grandfather of the author Robert Louis Stevenson, completed his 115 feet high lighthouse in 1811. This arguably most formidable of all lighthouse locations is the site of the oldest sea-swept lighthouse off the British coast.

It may be possible to launch at St. Andrews but, surprisingly, there are no launching facilities at Arbroath harbour, although it is possible to hire a trawler there. It may also be possible to launch at the old ferry slips at Dundee or Tayport.

THE TAY & ARBROATH

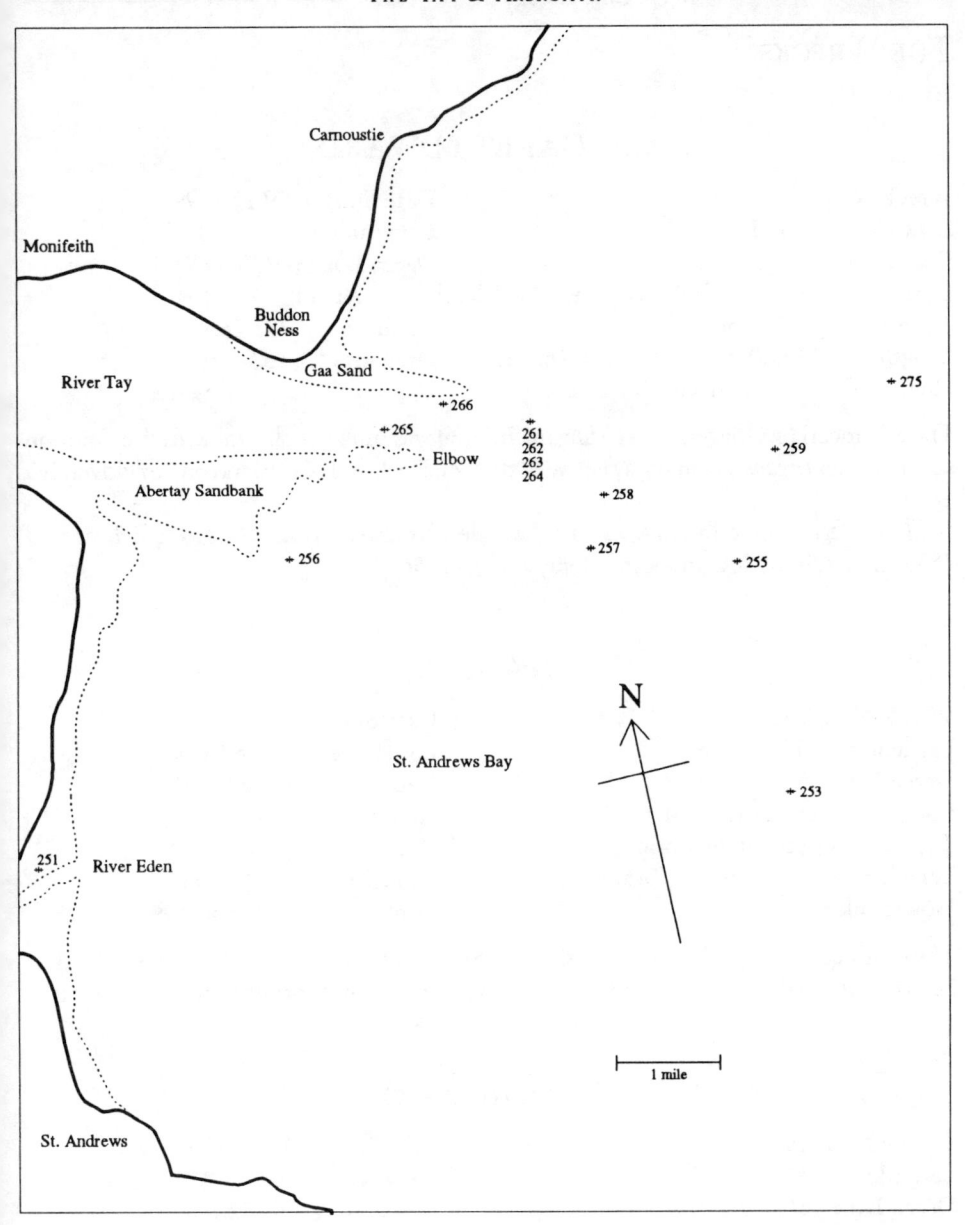

Chart of the wrecks lying off the mouth of the River Tay

The Wrecks

MARGARET EDWARD

Wreck No : 250
Latitude : 56 21 00 N PA
Decca Lat : 5621.00 N
Location : Between Bell Rock and May Island
Type : Schooner ?
Length : 141.0 feet Beam : 26.9 feet
How Sunk : Collision with *Bredalbane*

Date Sunk : 09 11 1899
Longitude : 02 35 00 W PA
Decca Long : 0235.00 W
Area : Tay
Tonnage : 296 gross
Draught : 16.5 feet
Depth : metres

The Aberdeen jury-rigged vessel *Margaret Edward* was sunk in collision with the Granton steam trawler *Bredalbane* mid way between the Bell Rock and May Island on 9th November 1899.

Lloyds Register describes the vessel as "wooden 3-masted Tow.Lr." (towing lighter ?) of 253 tons net, built at Garmouth, Morayshire in 1856.

UNKNOWN

Wreck No : 251
Latitude : 56 22 54 N
Decca Lat : 5622.90 N
Location : St. Andrews Bay
Type : Broken platform
Length : feet Beam : feet
How Sunk :

Date Sunk :
Longitude : 02 48 51 W
Decca Long : 0248.85 W
Area : Tay
Tonnage :
Draught : feet
Depth : metres

The obstruction charted close to the shore in St. Andrews Bay at 562254N, 024851W has been reported to be a "broken platform". (No mention was made of any train standing at it!).

UGIE (POSSIBLY)

Wreck No : 252
Latitude : 56 22 59 N
Decca Lat : 5622.98 N
Location : St. Andrews Bay
Type : Steamship
Length : 130.0 feet Beam : 21.1 feet
How Sunk :

Date Sunk : 16 03 1900
Longitude : 02 27 40 W
Decca Long : 0227.67 W
Area : Tay
Tonnage : 236 gross
Draught : 10.0 feet
Depth : 27 metres

A wreck about 42 metres long (138.6 feet), lying 109/289°, was first reported in this position on 7/12/1976.

This may be the Ugie (ex-*Reine des Belges*, ex-*Piscator*), an iron screw steamship of 236 tons gross, 130.0 x 21.1 x 10.0 feet, built in 1886 by McKnight of Ayr, engined by Muir & Houston, Glasgow.

The *Bodo*, for which an accurate position is unknown, was 139.3 feet long.

SOPHRON

Wreck No :	253	Date Sunk :	22 08 1917
Latitude :	56 23 30 N	Longitude :	02 35 45 W
Decca Lat :	5623.50 N	Decca Long :	0235.75 W
Location :	Off St. Andrews	Area :	Tay
Type :	Trawler	Tonnage :	195 gross
Length :	113.6 feet Beam : 21.0 feet	Draught :	11.2 feet
How Sunk :	Mined	Depth :	24 metres

The *Sophron* was a steel screw ketch (steam trawler) built in 1903 by Cook, Welton & Gemmell of Hull, and registered in Grimsby.

The 1919 position given for her sinking was 562335N, 023530W PA. In 1970 Alex Crawford located a wreck at 562330N, 023545W very close to the approximate position given for the *Sophron* in 1919.

The wreck found lies in about 24 metres, with lots of net over bow and stern, making identification very difficult. Alex Crawford suggested that it might be a submarine, but in that same year, he also suggested that the 400 feet long wreck at 562735N, 023218W, which is most likely to be the 5548 tons gross steamship *Nailsea River*, may have been a submarine. Was Captain Crawford perhaps looking for a submarine that year?

Great respect is due to Alex Crawford for his salvage of the liner *Oceanic* off Foula, Shetland, and the cruiser HMS *Argyll* off the Bell Rock.

TORDENSKJOLD

Wreck No :	254	Date Sunk :	23 10 1881
Latitude :	56 15 00 N PA	Longitude :	02 48 00 W PA
Decca Lat :	5625.00 N	Decca Long :	0248.00 W
Location :	Kinshaldy Sands	Area :	Tay
Type :	Barque	Tonnage :	471 gross
Length :	136.0 feet Beam : 30.0 feet	Draught :	16.6 feet
How Sunk :	Ran aground	Depth :	metres

Tordenskjold was a Norwegian barque of 178 tons net, built in 1864 and registered in Drammen. She was lost on Kinshaldy Sands on 23rd October 1881.

UC-41

Wreck No :	255	Date Sunk :	21 08 1917
Latitude :	56 25 44 N	Longitude :	02 36 27 W
Decca Lat :	5625.74 N	Decca Long :	0236.46 W
Location :	Mouth of the Tay	Area :	Tay
Type :	Submarine	Tonnage :	417 disp.
Length :	163.0 feet Beam : 17.2 feet	Draught :	12.2 feet
How Sunk :		Depth :	23 metres

This wreck was first recorded on 31st January 1934 at 562548N 023622W. It is in two parts, one 100 feet long *, lying 037/217°, the other not more than 50 feet long close North of the centre of the larger part.

It was dived in 1989 at 562544N 023628W and recognised as a UC2 class mine laying U-Boat in two sections 20 metres apart, in a depth of 27 metres.

UC-41 (Foerste) was sunk in an accident with her own mines on 21st August 1917, in or off the Tay estuary. (It has also been suggested that she was sunk by the trawlers *Jacinta*, *Thomas Young* and *Chirkara*).

UC-41 displaced 417 tons on the surface, 493 tons submerged.

* The length of this longer part was actually recorded as about 200 feet, but I assume this must be a transcription error, as UC-41 was only 163 feet long.

STANCOURT

Wreck No :	256	Date Sunk :	30 01 1940
Latitude :	56 25 52 N	Longitude :	02 44 22 W
Decca Lat :	5625.87 N	Decca Long :	0244.37 W
Location :	Mouth of the Tay	Area :	Tay
Type :	Steamship	Tonnage :	956 gross
Length :	215.0 feet Beam : 31.5 feet	Draught :	13.8 feet
How Sunk :	Ran aground	Depth :	1 metres

The wreck charted at 562552N, 024422W is visible at low water, and was in this position near the South East edge of Abertay sands on 13/8/1943.

The *Stancourt* (ex-*Oder*), was built in 1909 by Ramage & Ferguson of Leith.

She was attacked by aircraft on 30/1/1940 and sustained serious bomb damage, and was run ashore on Abertay sands, but the wreck was subsequently recovered, (date unknown), and taken South for repair. (To Leith?).

FERTILE VALE

Wreck No :	257	Date Sunk :	17 07 1941
Latitude :	56 26 10 N	Longitude :	02 39 18 W
Decca Lat :	5626.17 N	Decca Long :	0239.30 W
Location :	Off the Tay	Area :	Tay
Type :	Drifter	Tonnage :	91 gross
Length :	feet Beam : feet	Draught :	feet
How Sunk :	Collision	Depth :	metres

Fertile Vale (ex-*Fogbow*), was a drifter built in 1917 and requisitioned for Admiralty use in December 1939. She sank in a collision off the Tay on 17/7/1941.

CLAN SHAW

Wreck No :	258	Date Sunk :	23 01 1917
Latitude :	56 26 28 N	Longitude :	02 38 43 W
Decca Lat :	5626.47 N	Decca Long :	0238.72 W
Location :	Mouth of the Tay	Area :	Tay
Type :	Steamship	Tonnage :	3943 gross
Length :	360.0 feet Beam : 48.1 feet	Draught :	24.5 feet
How Sunk :	Mined	Depth :	8 metres

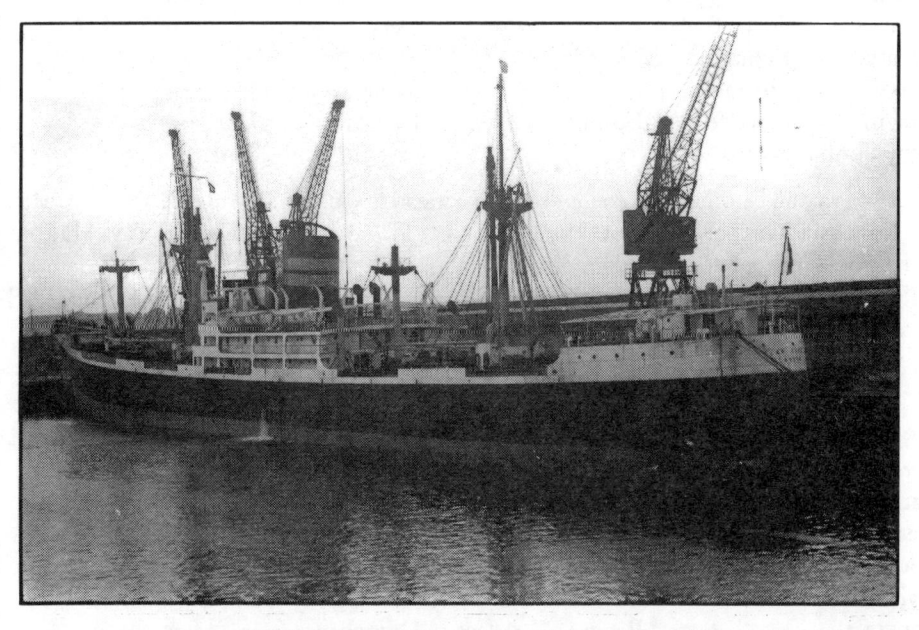

Clan Shaw (photograph reproduced with the permission of Glasgow University Archives)

Clan Shaw was a steel screw steamer built in 1902 by W. Doxford & Sons Ltd., Sunderland, and registered in Glasgow.

Two lives were lost when she was mined in the mouth of the Tay on 23/1/1917. Because of the size of the vessel and the shallow depth, part of her hull and superstructure remained visible above the surface for a time after she settled on the bottom, making her position relatively easy to establish with accuracy, and she was charted at 562632N, 023846W.

Either the shifting sands have moved the wreck slightly over the years, or her position was not recorded quite as accurately as it might have been, as she was relocated close by at 562628N, 023843W in 1955.

The wreck was reported to be apparently intact and approximately 200 feet long in a general depth of 10 metres. It is now charted as 7.9 metres on the 10 metre contour off the Abertay sand bank, but depths in this area vary with movements of the sand due to tidal action. Wreckage probably covers and uncovers, but is mostly buried, accounting for the discrepancy in the reported length of the wreck as approximately 200 feet, versus the 360 feet actual length of the *Clan Shaw*.

It was dived in 1989 and described as an incomplete large wreck in 15 metres to a muddy seabed. The stern stood up 3 metres from the bottom. It seemed to have been dispersed, as the forward part was apparently missing.

ANU

Wreck No :	259	Date Sunk :	06 02 1940
Latitude :	56 26 54 N	Longitude :	02 35 41 W
Decca Lat :	5626.90 N	Decca Long :	0235.68 W
Location :	Mouth of the Tay	Area :	Tay
Type :	Steamship	Tonnage :	1421 gross
Length :	250.0 feet Beam : 36.2 feet	Draught :	17.6 feet
How Sunk :	Mined	Depth :	20 metres

The *Anu* was an Estonian coaster built by J. Redhead & Co. in 1883, mined and sunk with the loss of six lives between Nos. 2 and 1 buoys at the entrance to the river Tay, while en route from Gothenburg and Aberdeen to Dundee with a cargo of paper.

She was located in 1969, lying 045/225° with a least depth of 65 feet in 70 feet, embedded in a sandy bottom.

CALCEOLARIA

Wreck No :	260	Date Sunk :	27 10 1918
Latitude :	56 27 00 N PA	Longitude :	02 40 00 W PA
Decca Lat :	5627.00 N	Decca Long :	0240.00 W
Location :	Off Elbow Light Buoy	Area :	Tay
Type :	Drifter	Tonnage :	92 gross
Length :	feet Beam : feet	Draught :	feet

How Sunk :	Mined	Depth :	metres

The hired drifter *Calceolaria* was mined off the Elbow light buoy on 27th October 1918.

The wreck of a small trawler type vessel, standing on an even keel about 3 metres above the sand, has been found at 562706N 023548W. This could be the *Calceolaria*, *Ben Ardna*, *Frons Oliviae*, *Girl Eva* or *Lena Melling*.

Depth to the top of the wreck is 25 metres, while depth to the sandy seabed is 28 metres.

BEN ARDNA

Wreck No :	261	Date Sunk :	08 08 1915
Latitude :	56 27 00 N PA	Longitude :	02 40 00 W PA
Decca Lat :	5627.00 N	Decca Long :	0240.00 W
Location :	Off the Elbow Buoy	Area :	Tay
Type :	Trawler	Tonnage :	197 gross
Length :	feet Beam : feet	Draught :	feet
How Sunk :	Mined	Depth :	metres

The *Ben Ardna* was an Aberdeen trawler requisitioned for use as a mine sweeper in the first world war. She hit a mine and sank off the Elbow Buoy on 8th August 1915. Elbow Buoy is at 562709N, 024040W in the mouth of the Tay, marking the shipping channel.

There is very shallow water in this area of shifting sand banks. Any wrecks here are likely to be buried in the sand.

FRONS OLIVIAE

Wreck No :	262	Date Sunk :	12 10 1915
Latitude :	56 27 00 N PA	Longitude :	02 40 00 W PA
Decca Lat :	5627.00 N	Decca Long :	0240.00 W
Location :	Off the Elbow Buoy	Area :	Tay
Type :	Drifter	Tonnage :	98 gross
Length :	feet Beam : feet	Draught :	feet
How Sunk :	Mined	Depth :	metres

The hired drifter *Frons Oliviae* was mined off the Elbow buoy on 12th October 1915.

GIRL EVA

Wreck No :	263	Date Sunk :	02 10 1916
Latitude :	56 27 00 N PA	Longitude :	02 40 00 W PA
Decca Lat :	5627.00 N	Decca Long :	0240.00 W
Location :	Off the Elbow Buoy	Area :	Tay

Type :	Drifter			Tonnage :	76 gross
Length :		feet	Beam :	feet	Draught :		feet
How Sunk :	Mined			Depth :		metres

The hired drifter *Girl Eva* was mined off the Elbow light buoy on 2nd October 1916.

LENA MELLING

Wreck No :	264			Date Sunk :	23 04 1916
Latitude :	56 27 00 N PA			Longitude :	02 40 00 W PA
Decca Lat :	5627.00 N			Decca Long :	0240.00 W
Location :	Near the Elbow Buoy			Area :	Tay
Type :	Trawler			Tonnage :	274 gross
Length :	125.0 feet	Beam :	23.5 feet	Draught :	12.8 feet
How Sunk :	Mined			Depth :	0 metres

The hired trawler *Lena Melling* was mined near the Elbow light buoy on 23rd April 1916. She was a steel screw ketch built by Smiths Dock, Middlesbrough in 1915.

SUTLEJ

Wreck No :	265			Date Sunk :	31 03 1858
Latitude :	56 27 00 N PA			Longitude :	02 42 30 W PA
Decca Lat :	5627.00 N			Decca Long :	0242.50 W
Location :	4.5 miles E of Tentsmuir Point			Area :	Tay
Type :	Steamship			Tonnage :	782 gross
Length :	feet	Beam :	feet	Draught :	feet
How Sunk :				Depth :	16 metres

This position is mid way between Nos. 1 and 2 Navigation Buoys, Elbow End. The general depth in the area is 16 metres to a sandy bottom.

PROTECTOR

Wreck No :	266	Date Sunk :	1889
Latitude :	56 27 25 N	Longitude :	02 41 34 W
Decca Lat :	5627.42 N	Decca Long :	0241.57 W
Location :	Gaa Sand, 1 mile E of Buddon	Area :	Tay
Type :	Paddle Tug	Tonnage :	89 gross

Length :	89.3 feet	Beam : 18.0 feet	Draught :	9.5 feet	
How Sunk :			Depth :	8 metres	

The wreck of the paddle tug *Protector* is charted 4.5 miles East of Tentsmuir Point, and 1.5 miles from Old Low Lighthouse which is on Buddon Ness between Carnoustie and Monifieth.

UNKNOWN

Wreck No :	267		Date Sunk :	
Latitude :	56 21 46 N		Longitude :	02 12 12 W
Decca Lat :	5621.77 N		Decca Long :	0212.20 W
Location :	7.5 miles SE of Bell Rock		Area :	Arbroath
Type :			Tonnage :	
Length :	feet	Beam : feet	Draught :	feet
How Sunk :			Depth :	49 metres

Charted as Wk 49 metres in 55 metres, 7.5 miles South East of the Bell Rock.

UNKNOWN

Wreck No :	268		Date Sunk :	
Latitude :	56 22 40 N		Longitude :	02 16 48 W
Decca Lat :	5622.67 N		Decca Long :	0216.80 W
Location :	5 miles SE of Bell Rock		Area :	Arbroath
Type :			Tonnage :	
Length :	feet	Beam : feet	Draught :	feet
How Sunk :			Depth :	51 metres

Charted as Wk 51 metres in 54 metres, 5 miles South East of the Bell Rock. The date of first reporting this wreck is not known, but it might be the *Margaret Edward*, sunk in collision with the Granton steamer *Bredalbane*, mid way between the Bell Rock and May Island on 9th November 1899.

HERRINGTON

Wreck No :	269		Date Sunk :	04 05 1917
Latitude :	56 37 12 N		Longitude :	02 37 36 W
Decca Lat :	5637.20 N		Decca Long :	0237.60 W
Location :	3/4 mile E of Red Head		Area :	Arbroath

Type :	Steamship		Tonnage :	1258 gross	
Length :	230.5 feet	Beam : 36.0 feet	Draught :	14.9 feet	
How Sunk :	Mined		Depth :	22 metres	

The 1258 ton collier Herrington was a steel screw steamship built in 1905 by S.P. Austin of Sunderland, engined by Richardsons, Westgarth & Co., Sunderland.

She was mined on 4th May 1917. The position was originally described as ³/₄ mile ESE of Red Head, Forfar, but the wreck is charted as ³/₄ mile East of Red Head. (This may be due to the effect of the change in the magnetic variation since 1917).

The *Herrington* had sailed from Methil with a cargo of coal. The mine she hit had been laid by the *UC-77*.

The wreck has been found in 30 metres of water, lying on a rocky bottom at 573712N 022736W. Least depth to the wreck is 20 metres.

The wreck is complete but not intact. The forward section, from the bow to the boilers is upside down, while the after section from the engines to the stern is lying over on its port side. There is one boiler and a three-cylinder engine. Cutlery found bears the inscription *Herrington*.

UNKNOWN

Wreck No :	270		Date Sunk :	
Latitude :	56 23 00 N		Longitude :	02 16 36 W
Decca Lat :	5623.00 N		Decca Long :	0216.60 W
Location :	5 miles SE of Bell Rock		Area :	Arbroath
Type :			Tonnage :	
Length :	feet	Beam : feet	Draught :	feet
How Sunk :			Depth :	40 metres

Charted as Wk 40 metres in 51 metres, 5 miles South East of the Bell Rock.

BRACONBURN

Wreck No :	271		Date Sunk :	30 07 1944
Latitude :	56 25 00 N PA		Longitude :	02 20 00 W PA
Decca Lat :	5625.00 N		Decca Long :	0220.00 W
Location :	Near the Bell Rock		Area :	Arbroath
Type :	Trawler		Tonnage :	203 gross
Length :	feet	Beam : feet	Draught :	feet
How Sunk :	Collision		Depth :	metres

Braconburn (ex-*Richard Briscoll*) was a steam trawler built in 1918 by Duthie of Aberdeen. In 1944 she was requisitioned for use as a blockship, and was en route to Scapa Flow when she was sunk near the Bell Rock in collision with the liberty ship *Le Baron Russell Briggs* on 30/7/1944. Six crew members were lost. The lat/long given at the time was 56 35 00 N 02 10 00 W. No wreck is in that position but the 200 ft long by 15 ft high wreck at 56 37 24 N 02 09 06 W may be the *Braconburn*.

Le Baron Russell Briggs was scuttled in 16000 feet of water 283 miles off Cape Kennedy, Florida on 18th August 1970, with a cargo of lethal nerve gas.

UNKNOWN

Wreck No :	272	Date Sunk :	
Latitude :	56 25 06 N	Longitude :	02 14 00 W
Decca Lat :	5625.10 N	Decca Long :	0214.10 W
Location :	5 miles E of Bell Rock	Area :	Arbroath
Type :		Tonnage :	
Length : feet	Beam : feet	Draught :	feet
How Sunk :		Depth :	49 metres

Charted as Wk 49 metres in 56 metres, 5 miles East of the Bell Rock. Possibly the *Braconburn?*

ARGYLL

Wreck No :	273	Date Sunk :	28 10 1915
Latitude :	56 26 00 N	Longitude :	02 23 30 W

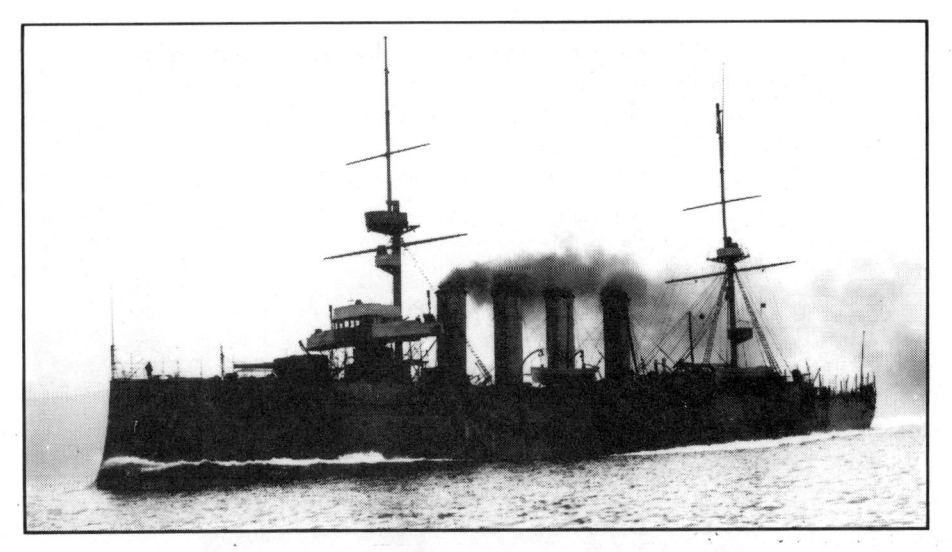

HMS Argyll (photograph reproduced with the permission of Glasgow University Archives)

Decca Lat :	5626.00 N		Decca Long :	0223.50 W
Location :	W. side of Bell Rock		Area :	Arbroath
Type :	Cruiser		Tonnage :	10850 gross
Length :	450.0 feet	Beam : 68.5 feet	Draught :	25.5 feet
How Sunk :	Ran aground		Depth :	15 metres

The cruiser HMS *Argyll* ran on to the Bell Rock during the night while the lighthouse was blacked out.

Extensive salvage has been carried out, and the remains are now well broken up and scattered in fairly shallow water on the West side of the reef, about 420 feet West of the lighthouse. Despite the salvage work, there are still worthwhile non-ferrous goodies to be found, including portholes, but beware of shells for the large-calibre guns. The propellers have gone, but the huge shafts are still there.

QUIXOTIC

Wreck No :	274		Date Sunk :	05 12 1939
Latitude :	56 26 00 N		Longitude :	02 23 00 W
Decca Lat :	5626.00 N		Decca Long :	0223.00 W
Location :	Bell Rock		Area :	Arbroath
Type :	Trawler		Tonnage :	197 gross
Length :	feet	Beam : feet	Draught :	feet
How Sunk :	Ran aground		Depth :	metres

The steam trawler *Quixotic*, built 1898, ran on to the Bell Rock in darkness, immediately under the lighthouse, which was not lit because of the blackout imposed during the war. The lighthouse keepers threw ropes which the crew of the *Quixotic* were unable to reach. The crew then set fire to their bedding to act as flares which were seen on the mainland, and the Arbroath and Broughty Ferry lifeboats went out. The Broughty Ferry boat was able to approach close enough for the nine crew to jump aboard.

NAILSEA RIVER

Wreck No :	275		Date Sunk :	15 09 1940
Latitude :	56 27 35 N		Longitude :	02 32 18 W
Decca Lat :	5627.58 N		Decca Long :	0232.30 W
Location :	6 miles S of Arbroath		Area :	Arbroath
Type :	Steamship		Tonnage :	5548 gross
Length :	410.2 feet	Beam : 52.2 feet	Draught :	30.2 feet
How Sunk :	Aircraft torpedo		Depth :	24 metres

In 1969 HMS *Beagle* found a low wreck about 380 feet long lying 298/128° almost buried in sand, but giving a good sonar echo from all directions.

An indication of how little of this wreck remained unburied may be gained from the reported least depth of 81 feet in 82 feet. Alex Crawford dived on this wreck in November 1970 and thought it could possibly be a submarine, although he estimated its length to be about 400 feet, and reported it to be well silted up in a seabed of sand and mud.

In 1971 a suggestion was made that this might possibly be the *UC-41*, but the length dimension given by Alex Crawford and HMS *Beagle* does not coincide with *UC-41*, which was only 163 feet long, 17.2 feet beam, 12.2 feet draught, and weighed 417 tons on the surface, 493 tons submerged.

UC-41 (Foerste) was lost in an accident with its own mines in, (or off), the Tay estuary on 21st August 1917 and is at 562544N 023628W.

The only vessel known to have been lost in this area which closely matches the length of this wreck is the *Nailsea River* (ex-*Actor*), a 410 feet long, 5548 tons gross British steamship built in 1917 by D & W Henderson of Glasgow, and operated by Manchester Lines. At 22.30 hrs on 15th September 1940, while en route from Buenos Aires to the Tyne with a cargo of 7000 tons of wheat, she was reported to have been attacked 4 miles East of Montrose by a torpedo-carrying aircraft of the same enemy formation which had sunk the *Halland* shortly before.

She may have foundered here while attempting to reach Dundee after the attack.

BAY FISHER

Wreck No : 276	Date Sunk : 07 02 1941
Latitude : 56 28 09 N	Longitude : 02 19 12 W
Decca Lat : 5628.15 N	Decca Long : 0219.20 W
Location : 3.5 miles NE of Bell Rock	Area : Arbroath
Type : Steamship	Tonnage : 575 gross
Length : 164.8 feet Beam : 27.0 feet	Draught : 11.1 feet
How Sunk : Bombed	Depth : metres

Built in 1919 by J. Lewis & Son, Aberdeen, the 575 ton steamship *Bay Fisher* was bombed at 11.00 hrs on 7th February 1941. Four survivors were picked up by HMS *Heliopolis* and taken to Dundee.

HOCHE

Wreck No : 277	Date Sunk : 29 10 1915
Latitude : 56 30 16 N	Longitude : 02 36 30 W
Decca Lat : 5630.27 N	Decca Long : 0236.60 W
Location : Off Arbroath	Area : Arbroath

Type :	Sailing ship	Tonnage :	2211 gross
Length :	276.6 feet Beam : 40.3 feet	Draught :	22.5 feet
How Sunk :		Depth :	20 metres

This wreck was first located in 1969, and is about 300 feet long, standing up 15 feet in a general depth of 21 metres, lying NE/SW.

It may be the *Hoche*, or possibly the similarly-sized *Cerne*.

The *Hoche* was a French sailing ship built at Nantes in 1901.

CERNE

Wreck No :	278	Date Sunk :	26 03 1916
Latitude :	56 30 21 N PA	Longitude :	02 36 24 W PA
Decca Lat :	5630.35 N	Decca Long :	0236.40 W
Location :	4 miles NE of Elbow Buoy	Area :	Arbroath
Type :	Steamship	Tonnage :	2579 gross
Length :	315.0 feet Beam : 45.0 feet	Draught :	22.5 feet
How Sunk :	Mined	Depth :	20 metres

According to *British Vessels Lost at Sea 1914-18*, the British steamship *Cerne* was mined 4 miles NE of Elbow buoy on 26/3/1916. She was built by S.P. Austin of Sunderland in 1915 and engined by S. Clarke & Co.

A wreck is charted as 19.2 metres at 563016N, 023630W although I believe 563021N 023624W is more accurate, and this coincides with the position described in 1916. It is most likely the *Cerne*, although it may possibly be the similarly-sized *Hoche*.

The complete wreck is still there. The bows are intact on the starboard side and the after section is partly buried in mud. Depth to the bow is 20 metres, while the muddy seabed is at 24 metres.

UNKNOWN - CANGANIAN?

Wreck No :	279	Date Sunk :	17 11 1916
Latitude :	56 35 24 N	Longitude :	02 21 30 W
Decca Lat :	5635.40 N	Decca Long :	0221.50 W
Location :	5 miles NE of Arbroath	Area :	Arbroath
Type :	Steamship	Tonnage :	1142 gross
Length :	227.7 feet Beam : 33.0 feet	Draught :	13.2 feet
How Sunk :	Foundered	Depth :	60 metres

This charted wreck, which lies NNW/SSE, was located on 15th September 1930 when the trawler *Camelia* fouled her gear.

It is apparently a large wreck, about 280 feet long, and standing up some 8 metres from the bottom in 62 metres.

The collier *Canganian* foundered 8-10 miles from Montrose on 17th November 1916 while en route from Methil to Scapa Flow, but this wreck is substantially longer than the *Canganian* which was 227.7 feet long.

The position has also been recorded as 563520N, 012130W.

LORD BEACONSFIELD

Wreck No :	280	Date Sunk :	17 10 1945
Latitude :	56 36 22 N	Longitude :	02 29 30 W
Decca Lat :	5636.37 N	Decca Long :	0229.50 W
Location :	Off Prail Castle, Auchmithie	Area :	Arbroath
Type :	Trawler	Tonnage :	302 gross
Length :	135.0 feet Beam : 23.5 feet	Draught :	12.3 feet
How Sunk :	Ran aground	Depth :	10 metres

The *Lord Beaconsfield* (ex-*Tribune*), was a hired Admiralty trawler, built in 1915 by Cochranes of Selby, engine by C.D. Holmes of Hull, and registered in Grimsby.

She ran aground almost under Prail Castle on 17th October 1945.

The ship's Walker log, engine room gauges and a Seibe Gorman diving knife with brass sheath have been recovered.

FOUNTAINS ABBEY

Wreck No :	281	Date Sunk :	15 11 1921
Latitude :	56 37 00 N PA	Longitude :	02 29 00 W PA
Decca Lat :	5637.00 N	Decca Long :	0229.00 W
Location :	Near Red Head	Area :	Arbroath
Type :	Steamship	Tonnage :	1285 gross
Length :	243.0 feet Beam : 32.2 feet	Draught :	18.0 feet
How Sunk :	Ran aground	Depth :	metres

The 1285 tons gross *Fountains Abbey* was a British steamship built in 1879 by Palmers Co., and registered in Leith.

She ran aground during the night of 15th November 1921 near Red Head, Forfar, between Arbroath and Montrose, while en route from Riga, Latvia, to Dundee with a cargo of flax and timber. The crew remained on the vessel until daybreak.

When the Arbroath and Montrose lifeboats arrived on the scene, the crew had already landed, with difficulty, on the rocky shore. The bottom of the hull of the *Fountains Abbey* was badly damaged, and later that morning she slipped off the rocks and sank. It was hoped that a considerable portion of her cargo could be salved before the wreck was broken up by tidal action.

CHAPTER 9

THE WRECKS OF MONTROSE, GOURDON & STONEHAVEN

INTRODUCTION

Sandy beaches in the southern part of this area give way to rocky shores towards the north. The rocky coast of Kincardineshire is relatively inaccessible from the land.

Montrose is almost surrounded by water at high tide; when the tide retreats it leaves the muddy expanse of Montrose Basin, which is a haunt of wildfowl. From Montrose there is a six mile stretch of sand backed by dunes and stretching to the small village of St. Cyrus.

There is a slip at Johnshaven, which is a small village some seven miles North of Montrose. The village is strung out along a ledge between the main road and a rocky beach.

Dramatic rough seas can be experienced around Gourdon during easterly gales because of the reefs which stretch almost a quarter of a mile out to sea. This village is situated on rocky slopes above its harbour where there are slipway launching facilities. Interestingly, it was the first Scottish fishing port to adapt motor boats for fishing in the early years of this century.

South of Stonehaven the sea has carved a series of small bays from sheer sandstone cliffs; some of these can be reached only by scrambling down rocky slopes.

Small inflatable boats can be launched across the stony beach at Catterline, a mile North of Tod Head, while larger boats can be launched from the slip at Stonehaven harbour.

Stonehaven nestles at the mouth of a sheltered valley formed by two rivers, the Carron Water and the Cowie Water. Fishing provided Stonehaven's initial prosperity (with some 120 vessels operating at the turn of the century) but, nowadays, the fishing boats are outnumbered by yachts and other pleasure craft.

Most of the diving in this area is from the shore, because the rapidly increasing depths offshore lead to wrecks being too deep for most sports divers. By comparison, many of the wrecks close to shore are well-broken due to the shallow water.

Aberdeen, 13 miles North of Stonehaven, is the nearest source of compressed air.

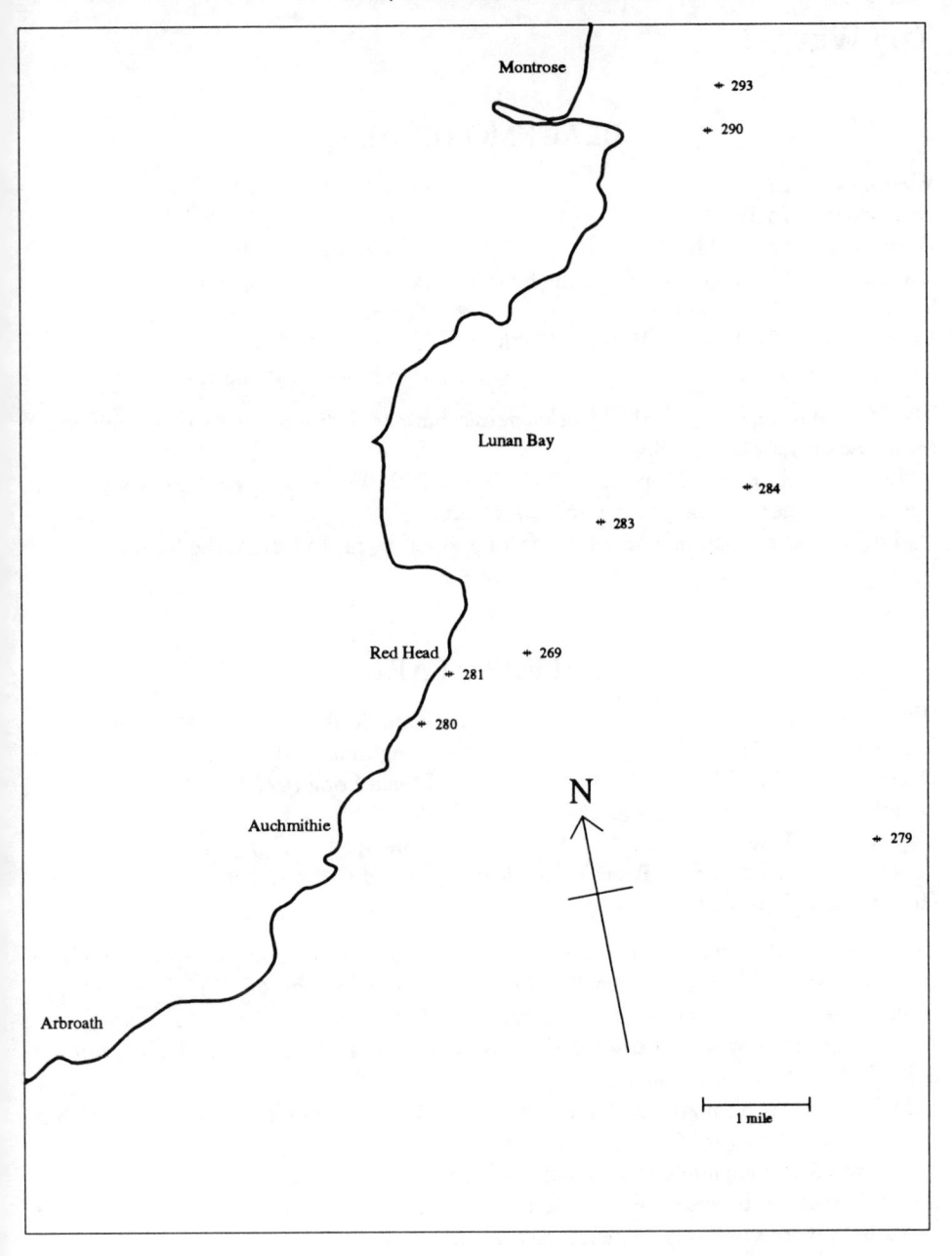

Chart of the wrecks lying between Auchmithie and Montrose

The Wrecks

BLACKMOREVALE

Wreck No :	282	Date Sunk :	01 05 1918
Latitude :	56 37 24 N	Longitude :	02 09 06 W
Decca Lat :	5637.40 N	Decca Long :	0209.10 W
Location :	10.5 miles SE of Scurdie Ness	Area :	Montrose
Type :	Mine sweeper	Tonnage :	750 gross
Length :	231.0 feet Beam : 28.0 feet	Draught :	7.0 feet
How Sunk :	Mined	Depth :	55 metres

The 750 ton mine sweeper HMS *Blackmorevale*, built at Ardrossan in 1916, was mined off Montrose on 1st May, 1918.

The wreck charted in 55 metres at 563724N, 010906W might be the *Blackmorevale*, but it is also considered to be possibly the *Braconburn*

This wreck is apparently about 200 ft long, standing up 15 ft from the bottom.

MILFORD EARL

Wreck No :	283	Date Sunk :	08 12 1941
Latitude :	56 38 42 N	Longitude :	02 23 48 W
Decca Lat :	5638.70 N	Decca Long :	0223.80 W
Location :	3 miles E of Lunan Bay	Area :	Montrose
Type :	Trawler	Tonnage :	290 gross
Length :	125.5 feet Beam : 23.5 feet	Draught :	12.7 feet
How Sunk :	By aircraft	Depth :	32 metres

The trawler *Milford Earl* (ex-*Duncan Mcrae*, ex-*Callancroft*, ex-*Andrew Apsley*), built in 1919 by Cook, Welton & Gemmell of Beverley, engine by Amos & Smith of Hull, was requisitioned for use as a mine sweeper in August 1939.

All 11 of the crew were lost when she was sunk 3 miles SE of Usan, by *HE111* aircraft of *KG26* from Stavanger, Norway.

In 1987, divers from Arbroath recovered an anti-aircraft gun from the wreck which is charted in 24 metres at 563842N, 022348W.

The wreck is completely intact, with a 20° list to port. There is a gun on the bow and depth charges on the stern. Shells dated 1918 have been found. Depth to the top of the wreck is 32 metres and it is 38 metres to the sandy seabed.

PHINEAS BEARD

Wreck No :	284	Date Sunk :	08 12 1941
Latitude :	56 38 45 N	Longitude :	02 26 06 W
Decca Lat :	5638.75 N	Decca Long :	0226.10 W
Location :	Lunan Bay, 4 miles S of Montrose	Area :	Montrose
Type :	Trawler	Tonnage :	278 gross
Length :	125.5 feet Beam : 23.5 feet	Draught :	12.7 feet
How Sunk :	By aircraft	Depth :	24 metres

The trawler *Phineas Beard* was built in 1918 by Cook, Welton & Gemmell of Hull, and requisitioned for use as a mine sweeper in August 1939.

Five of the crew were lost when she was sunk by aircraft off Lunan Bay, 1.5 miles North East of Red Head.

The wreck was charted at 563810N, 022700W, but has since been altered to 563824N, 022622W in 24 metres.

Position 563845N 022606W is, I believe, more accurate.

Although the midship section is damaged, the wreck is complete, with a 30° list to port. She is a steel-hulled trawler, armed with a gun on the bow. Shell cases dated 1940 have been found.

The least depth to the highest point of the wreck is 24 metres, while the depth to the sandy seabed is 30 metres.

ALMA

Wreck No :	285	Date Sunk :	20 09 1916
Latitude :	56 40 00 N PA	Longitude :	02 26 00 W PA
Decca Lat :	5640.00 N	Decca Long :	0226.00 W
Location :	Ashore at Lunan Bay	Area :	Montrose
Type :	Schooner	Tonnage :	335 gross
Length :	120.0 feet Beam : 28.7 feet	Draught :	14.0 feet
How Sunk :	Ran aground	Depth :	metres

The Danish 3-masted schooner *Alma* of Thuro, with a cargo of paper, was driven ashore at Lunan Bay near Montrose on 20th September 1916.

She was a wooden vessel built in 1893 by A. Buschman of Riga.

UNKNOWN - LH308 ?

Wreck No : 286
Latitude : 56 41 39 N
Decca Lat : 5641.65 N
Location : 10 miles E of Scurdy Ness Lighthouse.
Type :
Length :   feet   Beam :   feet
How Sunk :

Date Sunk : Pre-1929
Longitude : 02 07 30 W
Decca Long : 0207.50 W
Area :   Montrose
Tonnage :
Draught :   feet
Depth :   60 metres

First reported in 1929 and charted as Wk 60 metres. This may be the *Canganian*, or possibly the *Plethos*.

GREENAWN

Wreck No : 287
Latitude : 56 42 00 N PA
Decca Lat : 5642.00 N
Location : near Montrose
Type : Steamship
Length : 190.7 feet   Beam : 29.1 feet
How Sunk : Bombed?

Date Sunk : 03 04 1941
Longitude : 02 05 00 W PA
Decca Long : 0205.00 W
Area : Montrose
Tonnage : 784 gross
Draught : 11.9 feet
Depth :   metres

The 784 tons gross steamship *Greenawn* was built in 1924 by Hall of Aberdeen.

The cause of her loss near Montrose on 3rd April 1941 is unknown, but she is likely to have been bombed by German aircraft, as the 250 ton steamship *Cairnie* was bombed nearby on the same day, 6-8 miles S by W of Tod Head.

Another description given for the position of the *Cairnie* is 5 miles E of Johnshaven, while the Hydrographic Dept. has suggested she may have come ashore near Aberdeen on the 13th April.

H C GRUBE

Wreck No : 288
Latitude : 56 42 00 N PA
Decca Lat : 5642.00 N
Location : S end of Annat Bank, Montrose
Type : Schooner
Length : 115.7 feet   Beam : 26.1 feet
How Sunk : Ran aground

Date Sunk : 20 09 1916
Longitude : 02 26 00 W PA
Decca Long : 0226.00 W
Area : Montrose
Tonnage : 251 gross
Draught : 10.9 feet
Depth :   metres

The 3-masted steel schooner *H C Grube* of Marstal, Denmark, was driven on to the South end of Annat Bank at the entrance to Montrose harbour on 20th September 1916.
She was built in 1902 by Klippans of Gothenburg.

PLETHOS

Wreck No :	289		Date Sunk :	23 04 1918
Latitude :	56 42 00 N PA		Longitude :	02 05 00 W PA
Decca Lat :	5642.00 N		Decca Long :	0205.00 W
Location :	Off Montrose		Area :	Montrose
Type :	Trawler		Tonnage :	210 gross
Length :	115.0 feet	Beam : 22.6 feet	Draught :	12.1 feet
How Sunk :	Mined		Depth :	45 metres

The 210 tons gross steel screw ketch (steam trawler) *Plethos* was built in 1913 by A. Hall of Aberdeen, engine by W.V.V. Ligerwood of Glasgow.

She was requisitioned for use as a mine sweeper, and was mined off Montrose on 23rd April 1917.

CLINT

Wreck No :	290		Date Sunk :	15 03 1927
Latitude :	56 42 12 N		Longitude :	02 24 30 W
Decca Lat :	5642.20 N		Decca Long :	0224.50 W
Location :	1 mile E of Scurdyness Lighthouse.		Area :	Montrose
Type :	Steamship		Tonnage :	197 gross
Length :	125.0 feet	Beam : 20.0 feet	Draught :	9.0 feet
How Sunk :			Depth :	18 metres

Charted 1 mile E of Scurdy Ness lighthouse. She was a steel screw steamship built in 1896 by J. Fullerton of Paisley.

NORDHAV II

Wreck No :	291	Date Sunk :	10 03 1945
Latitude :	56 42 17 N	Longitude :	02 03 48 W
Decca Lat :	5642.28 N	Decca Long :	0203.80 W
Location :	Off Montrose	Area :	Montrose
Type :	Trawler	Tonnage :	425 gross

Length :   feet   Beam :   feet   Draught :   feet
How Sunk : Torpedoed by U-714   Depth :   metres

The Norwegian naval trawler *Nordhav II* was built in 1913, and requisitioned in 1940 as a mine sweeper.

She was sunk "off Dundee", 2 miles North of Buoy No. 25.

The Hydrographic Dept. gives 564230N, 020530W PA. The small wreck at 564217N, 020348W is the nearest accurate wreck position, and this could be the *Nordhav II*.

UNKNOWN - GREENAWN ?

Wreck No :   292   Date Sunk :
Latitude :   56 42 18 N   Longitude :   02 07 30 W
Decca Lat : 5642.30 N   Decca Long : 0207.50 W
Location :   12 miles E of Scurdy Ness Lighthouse.   Area :   Montrose
Type :   Tonnage :
Length :   feet   Beam :   feet   Draught :   feet
How Sunk :   Depth :   51 metres

Charted as Wk 51 metres. Possibly the *Greenawn* or the *Plethos*?

BEATHWOOD

Wreck No :   293   Date Sunk :   11 09 1940
Latitude :   56 42 36 N   Longitude :   02 24 18 W
Decca Lat : 5642.60 N   Decca Long : 0224.40 W
Location :   1 mile E Montrose CG Lookout   Area :   Montrose
Type :   Trawler   Tonnage :   209 gross
Length :   115.5 feet   Beam : 22.5 feet Draught :   12.4 feet
How Sunk :   Bombed   Depth :   16 metres

The steam trawler *Beathwood* (ex-*Osborne Stroud*), built in 1912 by A. Hall & Co., Aberdeen was bombed by German aircraft on 11th September 1940. She was in ballast at the time of sinking when 7 of the crew of 9 were lost.

There is a charted wreck 1 mile ENE of Scurdy Ness in 16 metres. My reading of the charted position is as given above, but another reference is 564236N, 022424W.

When dived, this was found to be the after section of a steel trawler, from the stern to the boiler. It is lying with a 45° list to port on a muddy seabed.

HEISTAD

Wreck No :	294	Date Sunk :	19 09 1916
Latitude :	56 43 00 N PA	Longitude :	02 26 00 W PA
Decca Lat :	5643.00 N	Decca Long :	0226.00 W
Location :	On Montrose Sands	Area :	Montrose
Type :	Schooner	Tonnage :	303 gross
Length :	124.9 feet Beam : 26.9 feet	Draught :	14.8 feet
How Sunk :	Ran aground	Depth :	metres

According to one source, the Norwegian 3-masted wooden schooner *Heistad*, with a cargo of pit props, was driven ashore on Montrose Sands on 19th September 1916.

Another report describes the vessel as a barque (incorrectly), en route from Porsgrund to the Tyne with pit props. In heavy seas, one of her crew was lost near the May Island on 19th November 1916, but that report suggests the vessel itself was not lost there at that time.

Presumably the crew member who was lost was washed overboard, and later that day the vessel was blown ashore on Montrose Sands.

The *Heistad* was built by Young of Prince Edward Island, Canada in 1874.

LETTIE

Wreck No :	295	Date Sunk :	09 11 1941
Latitude :	56 45 18 N PA	Longitude :	02 25 00 W PA
Decca Lat :	5645.30 N	Decca Long :	0225.00 W
Location :	Mouth of River Esk	Area :	Montrose
Type :	Tug	Tonnage :	89 gross
Length :	feet Beam : feet	Draught :	feet
How Sunk :	Ran aground	Depth :	metres

British Vessels Lost At Sea 1914-18 states HM Tug *Lettie* sunk, cause unknown, off St. Abbs Head, 9/11/1941. This is near the mouth of the river South Esk.

Another report states that an HM tug was driven ashore at the mouth of the North Esk, near Montrose the following day.

The previous report almost certainly refers to the *Lettie*, but a further report suggests the name of this vessel was *Buccaneer*, sunk by He-111s of the Luftwaffe while towing a battle practice target from Lunan Bay at 18.15 hrs on 9th November 1941, off Scurdy Ness. The crew of 43 were eventually rescued by breeches buoy.

PANSY

Wreck No :	296	Date Sunk :	11 12 1886
Latitude :	56 46 40 N PA	Longitude :	02 21 40 W PA
Decca Lat :	5646.67 N	Decca Long :	0221.67 W
Location :	Eastness, Burnmouth, St. Cyrus	Area :	Gourdon
Type :	Trawler	Tonnage :	
Length :	feet Beam : feet	Draught :	feet
How Sunk :	Ran aground	Depth :	metres

The South Shields steam trawler *Pansy* ran aground on the Eastness, Burnmouth, between St. Cyrus and Johnshaven on 11th December 1886.

UNKNOWN - U-Boat ?

Wreck No :	297	Date Sunk :	
Latitude :	56 47 12 N	Longitude :	02 11 48 W
Decca Lat :	5647.20 N	Decca Long :	0211.80 W
Location :	4 miles SE of Gourdon	Area :	Gourdon
Type :	Submarine ?	Tonnage :	
Length :	feet Beam : feet	Draught :	feet
How Sunk :		Depth :	51 metres

Charted as Wk 51 metres, 4.5 miles ESE of Johnshaven. The Hydrographic Dept. suggest this is a U-Boat, therefore the length should be about 160 - 200 feet

Could this be the *U-398*?

HAWNBY

Wreck No :	298	Date Sunk :	10 09 1914
Latitude :	56 47 42 N PA	Longitude :	02 19 00 W PA
Decca Lat :	5647.70 N	Decca Long :	0219.00 W
Location :	150 yards N of Johnshaven, Kincard.	Area :	Gourdon
Type :	Steamship	Tonnage :	2136 gross
Length :	280.0 feet Beam : 40.0 feet	Draught :	15.6 feet
How Sunk :	Ran aground	Depth :	8 metres

The 2136 tons gross steel steamship *Hawnby* was built in 1895 by R. Ropner & Son.

En route from Hull to Archangel with a cargo of coal and crew of 21, she ran aground on 10th September 1914. No lives were lost.

The position of stranding was originally reported as 150 yards North of Johnshaven, which is misleading, as that would put her inland, but she probably lies very close East of Johnshaven harbour.

Stonehaven
+ 313
+ 314

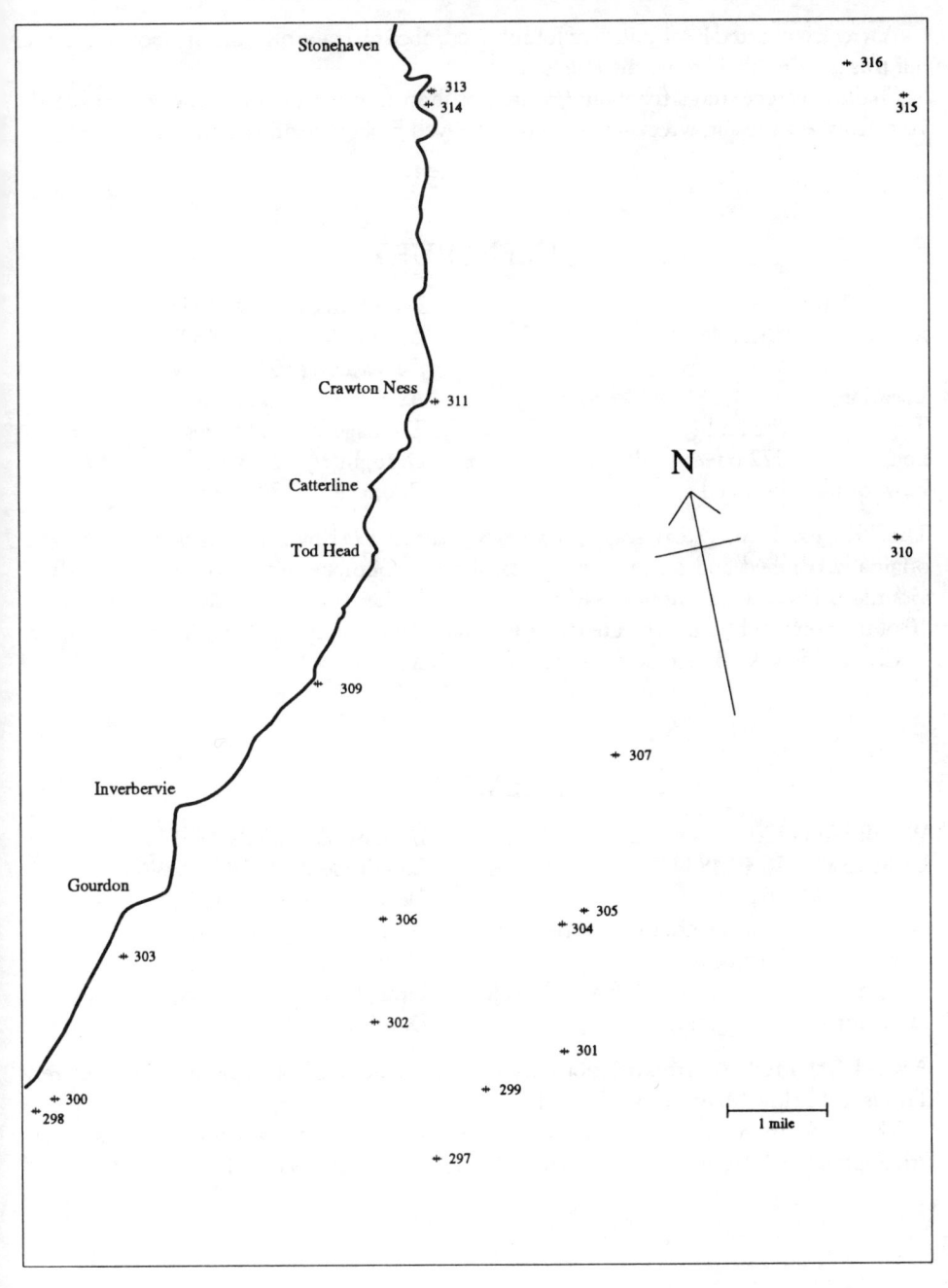

+ 316
+ 315

Crawton Ness
+ 311

Catterline

Tod Head

N

+ 310

+ 309

+ 307

Inverbervie

Gourdon
+ 305
+ 306
+ 304
+ 303

+ 302
+ 301

+ 300
+ 298
+ 299

1 mile

+ 297

Chart of the wrecks lying off the coast between Gourdon and Stonehaven

A wreck is charted PA 1 mile E of Johnshaven, about ¼ mile offshore, in about 8 metres, but this is more likely to be the *Balmoral*.

Shallow water extends for about ½ a mile offshore in this area, before the depth exceeds 10 metres. As a result, wreckage is likely to be well broken up and scattered.

QUEENSBURY

Wreck No :	299	Date Sunk :	06 06 1941
Latitude :	56 47 48 N	Longitude :	02 10 48 W
Decca Lat :	5647.80 N	Decca Long :	0210.80 W
Location :	4 miles SE of Gourdon	Area :	Gourdon
Type :	Steamship	Tonnage :	3911 gross
Length :	372.6 feet Beam : 52.3 feet	Draught :	24.4 feet
How Sunk :	Bombed	Depth :	50 metres

The 3911 ton British steamship *Queensbury*, built in 1931 by Burntisland S.B. Co., was originally bombed and set on fire and capsized by German aircraft 8 miles SE by E of Gourdon. There was no hope of saving the ship, which was sunk by convoy escort gunfire. 10 of the crew and 1 gunner were lost, the remainder being rescued by Montrose lifeboat.

Charted as Wk 50 metres, 5 miles E of Johnshaven.

BALMORAL

Wreck No :	300	Date Sunk :	09 09 1891
Latitude :	56 47 48 N PA	Longitude :	02 18 30 W PA
Decca Lat :	5647.80 N	Decca Long :	0218.50 W
Location :	Near Brotherton Castle, Kincard.	Area :	Gourdon
Type :	Steamship	Tonnage :	2045 gross
Length :	feet Beam : feet	Draught :	feet
How Sunk :	Ran aground	Depth :	8 metres

A wreck is charted PA in this position close to the shore, 1 mile E of Johnshaven, in 8 metres. This is just below Mains of Brotherton.

The 2045 ton iron steamship *Balmoral* was lost by stranding near Brotherton Castle on 9th September 1891, while en route from Chittagong to Dundee with a cargo of jute.

UNKNOWN - PRE 1940

Wreck No :	301	Date Sunk :	Pre-1940
Latitude :	56 47 50 N	Longitude :	02 09 36 W
Decca Lat :	5647.83 N	Decca Long :	0209.60 W
Location :	5 miles E of Johnshaven	Area :	Gourdon
Type :		Tonnage :	
Length : feet	Beam : feet	Draught :	feet
How Sunk :		Depth :	metres

Charted as a wreck with at least 28 metres over it in a general depth of 50 metres, 4.5 miles ESE of Gourdon. This wreck reportedly dates from pre-1940.

BAKU STANDARD

Wreck No :	302	Date Sunk :	11 02 1918
Latitude :	56 48 30 N	Longitude :	02 12 48 W
Decca Lat :	5648.50 N	Decca Long :	0212.80 W
Location :	4 miles E of Johnshaven	Area :	Gourdon
Type :	Tanker	Tonnage :	3708 gross
Length : 331.0 feet	Beam : 43.0 feet	Draught :	32.0 feet
How Sunk : Torpedoed		Depth :	40 metres

The 3708 tons gross tanker *Baku Standard* was built in 1903 by Armstrong Mitchell & Co.

She was torpedoed on 11th February 1918. *British Vessels Lost At Sea 1914-18* gives the position of the *Baku Standard* at the time of attack as 5 miles S by W $^1/_2$W from Tod Head. Twenty four of the crew were killed.

The wreck is charted at 564830N, 021248W, 2.5 miles SE of Gourdon, with a least depth of 34 metres in 44 metres.

SOAR

Wreck No :	303	Date Sunk :	18 03 1940
Latitude :	56 49 10 N PA	Longitude :	02 17 20 W PA
Decca Lat :	5649.17 N	Decca Long :	0217.33 W
Location :	1 mile S of Gourdon	Area :	Gourdon
Type :	Trawler	Tonnage :	219 gross
Length : feet	Beam : feet	Draught :	feet
How Sunk : Ran aground		Depth :	metres

The trawler *Soar* was returning to Aberdeen from a coaling trip to Methil on 18th March 1940 when she ran ashore on Black Waugh Rocks, 200 yards offshore, one mile South of Gourdon. The bodies of the six crewmen were washed ashore.

BELLONA II

Wreck No :	304	Date Sunk :	08 10 1940
Latitude :	56 49 24 N	Longitude :	02 09 30 W
Decca Lat :	5649.40 N	Decca Long :	0209.50 W
Location :	4 miles E of Gourdon, Kincard.	Area :	Gourdon
Type :	Steamship	Tonnage :	840 gross
Length :	feet Beam : feet	Draught :	feet
How Sunk :	Bombed	Depth :	46 metres

Charted as Wk PA with at least 28 metres over it in a general depth of 50 metres.
Another position which may be more accurate is 564932N, 020900W.

TAURUS

Wreck No :	305	Date Sunk :	06 06 1941
Latitude :	56 49 30 N PA	Longitude :	02 09 00 W PA
Decca Lat :	5649.50 N	Decca Long :	0209.00 W
Location :	4.5 miles E of Gourdon	Area :	Gourdon
Type :	Steamship	Tonnage :	4767 gross
Length :	408.0 feet Beam : 55.0 feet	Draught :	25.0 feet
How Sunk :	Bombed	Depth :	metres

The 4767 tons gross Norwegian steamship *Taurus*, en route from West Africa with 2000 tons of cocoa and 2000 tons of ground nuts was bombed by a German aircraft on 6th June 1941. She was taken in tow, but reportedly sank at 564925N, 020925W PA. Her crew were rescued by a drifter.

She could not be found there in 1967, but in 1976 the Board of Trade War Risks Department advised that she had been found, but no position was given.

She is now charted as a wreck in 48 metres at 564930N, 020900 PA.

UNKNOWN

Wreck No :	306	Date Sunk :	
Latitude :	56 49 30 N	Longitude :	02 12 36 W
Decca Lat :	5649.50 N	Decca Long :	0212.60 W
Location :	2.5 miles E of Gourdon	Area :	Gourdon
Type :		Tonnage :	
Length :	feet Beam : feet	Draught :	feet
How Sunk :		Depth :	40 metres

Charted as a wreck in about 40 metres.

REPRO

Wreck No : 307	Date Sunk : 26 04 1917
Latitude : 56 51 00 N	Longitude : 02 08 30 W
Decca Lat : 5651.00 N	Decca Long : 0208.50 W
Location : 4 miles E of Inverbervie	Area : Gourdon
Type : Trawler	Tonnage : 230 gross
Length : 117.3 feet Beam : 22.0 feet	Draught : 11.7 feet
How Sunk : Mined	Depth : metres

The 230 ton hired trawler (steel screw ketch) *Repro* was built in 1910 by Cook, Welton & Gemmell, engined by C.D. Holmes.

She was sunk by a mine on 23rd April 1917 and is charted as a wreck with at least 28 metres over it in a general depth of 44 metres, 3 miles SE of Tod Head lighthouse.

TANEVIK

Wreck No : 308	Date Sunk : 19 01 1945
Latitude : 56 51 48 N	Longitude : 01 55 42 W
Decca Lat : 5651.80 N	Decca Long : 0155.70 W
Location : 12 miles E of Gourdon	Area : Gourdon
Type :	Tonnage :
Length : feet Beam : feet	Draught : feet
How Sunk : Foundered in tow	Depth : 70 metres

Charted as Wk 70 metres, 11.5 miles E of Inverbervie.

The *Tanevik* was a balloon barrage vessel which foundered in tow from Methil to Buckie on 19th January 1945.

REINDEER

Wreck No : 309	Date Sunk : 19 11 1916
Latitude : 56 52 00 N PA	Longitude : 02 13 00 W PA
Decca Lat : 5652.00 N	Decca Long : 0213.00 W
Location : Off Shieldhill, Kincardineshire	Area : Stonehaven
Type : Steamship	Tonnage : 2412 gross
Length : 294.0 feet Beam : 43.1 feet	Draught : 17.2 feet
How Sunk : Ran aground	Depth : metres

The *Reindeer* was a steel screw steamship of 2412 tons gross, 1522 tons net, built in 1896 by J. Priestman, Sunderland, engine by T. Richardson of Hepple.

Her 20 crew were all lost when she stranded "off Shieldhill, Kincardineshire" while en route, in ballast, from Dieppe to Middlesbrough. Some wreckage was washed ashore at Todhead.

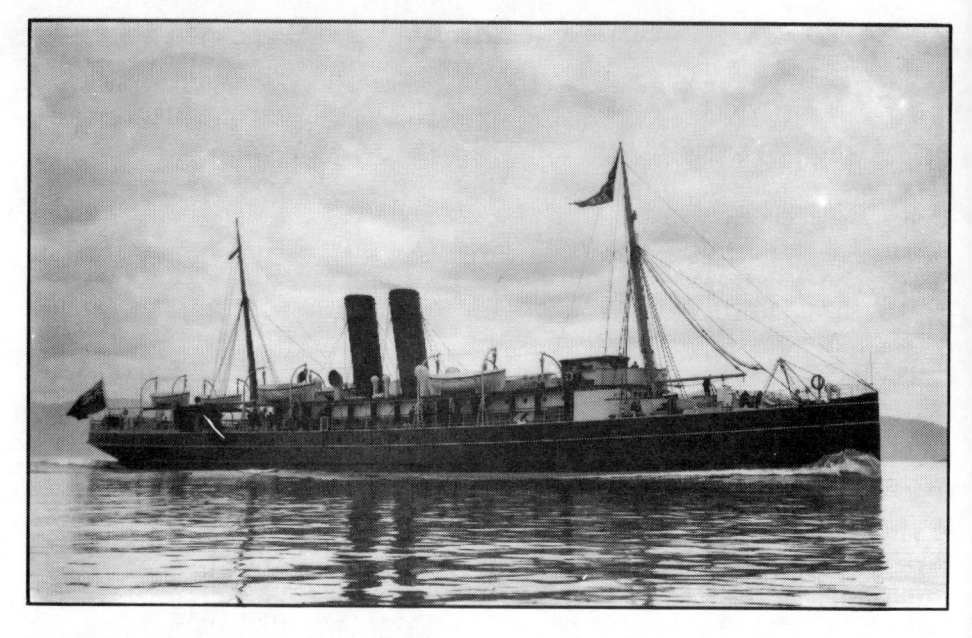

The Reindeer (photograph reproduced with the permission of Glasgow University Archives)

Kincardineshire is not on the direct route between Dieppe and Middlesbrough, but perhaps she was ordered to go by the scenic route around the North of Scotland, to avoid the Straits of Dover during the first world war.

Shieldhill is not identified on present day maps or charts, but it is at Whistleberry Castle.

The Hydrographic Dept. have recorded the *Reindeer* at 564932N, 020900W, which is several miles offshore, and hardly accords with running aground, but that position is almost identical to the charted position for the *Bellona II*.

UNKNOWN

Wreck No : 310		Date Sunk :	
Latitude : 56 53 04 N		Longitude : 02 03 12 W	
Decca Lat : 5653.07 N		Decca Long : 0203.20 W	
Location : 5 miles SE of Stonehaven		Area : Stonehaven	
Type :		Tonnage :	
Length : feet	Beam : feet	Draught :	feet
How Sunk :		Depth : 47 metres	

Charted 5.25 miles SE of Tod Head lighthouse, 4 miles E of Inverbervie.

GRANERO

Wreck No : 311		**Date Sunk :** 23 10 1933	
Latitude : 56 54 30 N		**Longitude :** 02 11 36 W	
Decca Lat : 5654.50 N		**Decca Long :** 0211.60 W	
Location : S side of Crawton Ness		**Area :** Stonehaven	
Type : Steamship		**Tonnage :** 1318 gross	
Length : 242.9 feet	**Beam :** 37.3 feet	**Draught :** 16.0 feet	
How Sunk : Ran aground		**Depth :** 16 metres	

The Norwegian steamship *Granero*, built in 1913, ran aground close to the shore at the South side of Crawton Ness, about three miles South of Stonehaven on 23rd October 1933.

The position has also been given as 562428N, 021118W.

While en route from Finland to Alloa with a cargo of pit props, she went on to the North side of the largest of the rocky fingers which stick out into Crawton Bay. This rocky promontory was used to mount the tripod for the breeches buoy during the rescue of the crew.

The wreck is now very broken up, with plates and girders strewn over a wide area. Maximum depth is 14-16 metres, but some of the plates have been moved into 3-6 metres, the wave action moving them like scythes, cutting down the kelp forest. The largest mass found so far is the chain locker and chain.

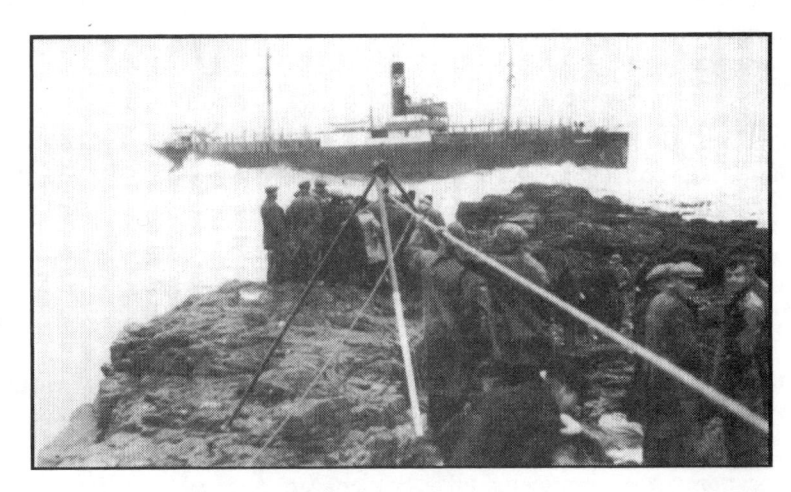

The Granero ashore at Crawton Ness in 1933 (photograph courtesy of City of Aberdeen, Arts Gallery and Museums Collections)

DESABLA

Wreck No :	312	Date Sunk :	12 06 1915
Latitude :	56 54 54 N	Longitude :	01 47 18 W
Decca Lat :	5654.90 N	Decca Long :	0147.30 W
Location :	13.5 miles ESE of Stonehaven	Area :	Stonehaven
Type :	Tanker	Tonnage :	6047 gross
Length :	420.3 feet Beam : 54.6 feet	Draught :	32.4 feet
How Sunk :	Torpedoed	Depth :	73 metres

Charted as a foul in about 73 metres. The 6047 tons gross tanker *Desabla*, built in 1913 by Hawthorn Leslie, was torpedoed 12 miles E of Tod Head on 12th June 1915 by the *U-17*.

Another report gives 15 miles E of Tod Head. She had been en route from Port Arthur, Texas, to the UK with a cargo of oil.

ECHO

Wreck No :	313	Date Sunk :	25 03 1928
Latitude :	56 57 18 N PA	Longitude :	02 11 45 W PA
Decca Lat :	5657.30 N	Decca Long :	0211.75 W
Location :	Strathlethan Bay, Stonehaven	Area :	Stonehaven
Type :	Steamship	Tonnage :	961 gross
Length :	230.0 feet Beam : 32.1 feet	Draught :	11.4 feet
How Sunk :	Ran aground	Depth :	metres

On 25th March 1928, the Norwegian steamship *Echo* ran ashore in fog at Strathlethan Bay, just to the South of Stonehaven, and became a total loss. She was built in 1891 by R. Dixon of Middlesbrough.

ISA FIORD

Wreck No :	314	Date Sunk :	19 09 1916
Latitude :	56 57 18 N PA	Longitude :	02 11 45 W PA
Decca Lat :	5657.30 N	Decca Long :	0211.75 W
Location :	At Strathlethan Bay, Stonehaven	Area :	Stonehaven
Type :		Tonnage :	
Length :	feet Beam : feet	Draught :	feet
How Sunk :	Ran aground	Depth :	metres

Wreckage from the Norwegian? vessel *Isa Fiord* of Koprevik was washed ashore at Strathlethan Bay, 1 mile South of Stonehaven on 19th September 1916.

GOWRIE

Wreck No :	315	Date Sunk :	09 01 1940
Latitude :	56 57 24 N	Longitude :	02 01 42 W
Decca Lat :	5657.40 N	Decca Long :	0201.70 W
Location :	5.5 miles E of Stonehaven	Area :	Stonehaven
Type :	Steamship	Tonnage :	689 gross
Length :	178.0 feet Beam : 30.0 feet	Draught :	12.3 feet
How Sunk :	Bombed	Depth :	54 metres

Charted as Wk 54 metres, the 689 ton steamship *Gowrie* was bombed and sunk en route from Hull to Aberdeen on 9th January 1940. Her crew of 12 were all saved.

CUSHENDALL

Wreck No :	316	Date Sunk :	29 06 1941
Latitude :	56 57 38 N	Longitude :	02 04 00 W
Decca Lat :	5657.63 N	Decca Long :	0204.00 W
Location :	4 miles E of Stonehaven	Area :	Stonehaven
Type :	Steamship	Tonnage :	626 gross
Length :	185.0 feet Beam : 27.6 feet	Draught :	10.8 feet
How Sunk :	Bombed	Depth :	46 metres

The 626 ton 3-masted steamship *Cushendall*, built in 1904 by Ailsa S.B. Co., Troon, engine by Muir & Houston, Glasgow, was bombed close off Stonehaven on 29th June 1941 at 5657N, 0203W.

She is now charted as a wreck in 46 metres at 565738N, 020400W.

MATADOR

Wreck No :	317	Date Sunk :	09 10 1924
Latitude :	56 59 22 N	Longitude :	02 04 24 W
Decca Lat :	5659.37 N	Decca Long :	0204.40 W
Location :	4.5 miles E of Stonehaven	Area :	Stonehaven
Type :	Steamship	Tonnage :	4761 gross
Length :	395.7 feet Beam : 51.5 feet	Draught :	26.7 feet
How Sunk :		Depth :	45 metres

Charted as a wreck in 45 metres, this may be the steamship *Matador*, sunk on 9th October 1924. The *Matador* (ex-*St. Veronica*, ex-*Arab*) was built in 1912 by J.L. Thompson of Sunderland.

CHAPTER 10

UNKNOWN WRECKS

O-13

Wreck No : 318		**Date Sunk :** 20 01 1940	
Latitude :		**Longitude :**	
Decca Lat :		**Decca Long :**	
Location : In the North Sea		**Area :** Unknown	
Type : Submarine		**Tonnage :** 568 gross	
Length : 198.5 feet **Beam :** 18.3 feet		**Draught :** 11.8 feet	
How Sunk : Torpedoed by *Wilk*		**Depth :** metres	

The Dutch submarine *O-13*, built by De Schelde in 1930, 468 tons surfaced, 715 tons submerged, powered by two Sulzer diesels and two electric motors, armed with five 21" torpedo tubes, (4 bow, 1 stern), and two 40 mm AA guns, had a crew of 31.

She was sunk in error "in the North Sea" by the Polish submarine *Wilk*. I suspect this may have occurred in the Southern North Sea, possibly off Heligoland, but could the *O-13* perhaps be the submarine reputedly sunk off Elie? (See the wreck at 560945N, 025045W).

The *Wilk*, built in France in 1929, escaped from the Baltic via the Sund Narrows, and arrived at Rosyth on 20/9/1939. She was used as a training ship from September 1940, based at HMS Ambrose, the Naval shore establishment at Dundee. Crew discipline was a serious problem, and Captain Krawcyk of the *Wilk* shot himself in the heart with his pistol immediately following a telephone call from London, in his office in HMS *Ambrose* at 15.00 hrs on 19th July 1941. Because of the poor condition of the *Wilk*, she was decommissioned on 2/4/1942, and was subsequently towed to Poland in 1951 for scrapping.

U-398

Wreck No :	319	Date Sunk :	05 1945
Latitude :		Longitude :	
Decca Lat :		Decca Long :	
Location :	Off East Coast of Scotland	Area :	Unknown
Type :	Submarine	Tonnage :	769 gross
Length :	221.4 feet Beam : 20.5 feet	Draught :	feet
How Sunk :	Unknown	Depth :	metres

U-398 was a Type VIIC U-Boat, 769 tons surfaced, 871 tons submerged. She was lost somewhere off the East coast of Scotland in May 1945.

ARCTURUS

Wreck No :	320	Date Sunk :	01 12 1939
Latitude :		Longitude :	
Decca Lat :		Decca Long :	
Location :	Off East Coast of Scotland	Area :	Unknown
Type :	Steamship	Tonnage :	1277 gross
Length :	229.9 feet Beam : 35.2 feet	Draught :	16.0 feet
How Sunk :	Torpedoed	Depth :	metres

The 1277 ton Norwegian steamship *Arcturus*, en route from Burntisland to Trondheim with a cargo of tea, gas stoves, steel wire cardboard folders, diaries, boots, shoes, and machinery, was sunk by a submarine off the East coast of Scotland on 1st December 1939. Nine of the crew were lost. Her position is unknown.

Appendix 1

Loss Analysis

Excluding those whose cause of loss is not known, and can therefore only be speculation, an analysis of the causes of loss of the vessels included in this book reveals the following:

Ran aground	127	51.8%	
Mined	31	12.7%	(Includes 1 trawling up a mine)
Collision	26	10.6%	
Foundered	17	6.9%	
By submarine	17	6.9%	(Includes torpedoes and gunfire)
By aircraft	17	6.9%	(Includes bombs, torpedoes and gunfire).
Scuttled	3	1.2%	
Fire/explosion	3	1.2%	(Includes 1 thought to have struck a mine)
Depth charged	2	0.8%	
Contact	1	0.4%	(Includes striking wreckage)
Rammed	1	0.4%	
Total war causes	69	28.1%	

It is interesting to compare the above statistics with *Lloyds Casualty Report* for 1991, which lists 258 ships of 100 tons gross and above, lost world-wide during that year. The total tonnage lost amounted to 1.5 million tons, and 1204 lives were lost, proving that modern technology has not eliminated shipping losses.

Foundered	111	43.0%	
Ran aground	45	17.4%	
Fire/explosion	37	14.3%	
Collision	36	14.0%	
War losses	13	5.0%	(Includes the Gulf War and Yugoslavia)
Contact	13	5.0%	
Missing	3	1.2%	

Lloyd's interpretation of *Contact* and my own may well be different, thus accounting for the discrepancy in figures in the tables.

Appendix 2

Diving information

Diving
A few words of caution might be appropriate for anyone contemplating diving in the Forth. Strong currents and tidal flow can be a serious problem in some places, and although this is not something which is peculiar to the Forth, it should be remembered that there is an awful lot of sea out there, and it is not unknown for divers to surface out of sight of the dive boat. Indeed, some divers have been lost. Helicopters and lifeboats have been called out, and fishing boats and other vessels in the area have had to be asked in the past to look for lost divers. This situation does not endear divers to the rescue services, or anyone else.

Boating
Crossing the shipping channels can sometimes seem like trying to cross a motorway. Apart from yachts and fishing trawlers, the river is used by many commercial vessels heading to and from the harbours of the Forth, and the Royal Navy operates ships into and out of Rosyth. Part of the area is designated as a submarine exercise area. There may, therefore, sometimes be submerged submarines.

Weather Information
H.M. Coastguard, (24 hours) for Berwick to Montrose; tel: Crail (0333) 50666
MARINECALL (24 hours); tel: 0898 500452. Provides a tape-recorded forecast, updated twice daily, for the area between Berwick and Rattray Head.

Dive centre
Les Pennington, East Coast Divers, West Pitkeirie, Anstruther; tel: Anstruther (0333) 310768
Air to 3200 psi, boat hire, bunkhouse accommodation for 15/16 divers.

Dive shops (air and equipment)
Edinburgh Diving Centre, 1, Watson Crescent, Edinburgh; tel: 031 229 4838
Hunter Diving, 44, Broughton Street, Edinburgh; tel: 031 556 5366

Air
Scoutscroft Diving Centre, Coldingham; tel: Coldingham (0890771) 338
Barefoots Caravan Park, Eyemouth; tel: Eyemouth (08907) 51050

Boat Charter
Ian Gatherum (MV *Aspire*); tel: Anstruther (0333) 730248
Jim Reaper (MV *Sapphire*); tel: Anstruther (0333) 310103
Russell Ritchie (MV *Guess Again*); tel: Anstruther (0333) 310697
Les Pennington; tel: Anstruther (0333) 310768

Appendix 3

Bibliography

The following is a list of publications and sources that were used for reference.

The Admiralty Hydrographic Department, Taunton.
All the World's Fighting Ships 1922-1946, pub. by Conway Maritime Press, 1980.
British Vessels Lost at Sea 1914-18 and 1939-45, pub. by Patrick Stephens, 1988
BSAC Wreck Register.
A Century of North Sea Passenger Steamers, by A. Greenaway, pub. Ian Allen 1986
Court of Enquiry Reports (various).
Dictionary of Disasters at Sea in the Age of Steam, by C. Hocking, pub. Lloyd's, 1989
Dive Scotland, Vol. III, by Gordon Ridley, pub. by Underwater World, 1992.
The Dundee Courier.
The Fife Free Press.
The Fifeshire Advertiser.
Guide to Diving in St. Abbs & Eyemouth Voluntary Marine Reserve, by C. Warman.
Jane's Book of Fighting Ships.
The K Boats, by Don Everitt, pub. by George G. Harrap, 1963.
Lloyds List of Shipping Losses.
Lloyds Register of Shipping.
Lloyds War Losses.
Parliamentary Papers (Various).
The Real Price of Fish, by George F Ritchie, pub. by Hutton Press, 1991.
Royal Naval Submarines 1901-1982, by M.P. Cocker, pub. by Frederick Warne.
The Scots Magazine, pub. by D.C. Thompson.
The Scotsman newspaper.
Shipwrecks Around Britain, by Leo Zanelli, pub. Kaye & Ward, 1970.
Steamers of the Forth, by Ian Brodie, pub. by David & Charles, 1976.
Submarines of World War 2, by Erminio Bagnasco pub. by Arms and Armour Press.
Unknown Shipwrecks Around Britain, by Leo Zanelli, pub. Kaye & Ward, 1974.
The U-Boat, by Eberhard Rossler pub. by Arms & Armour Press, 1981.
The U-Boat Offensive 1914-1945, by V.E. Tarrant, pub. by Arms & Armour Press, 1989.
Warship Losses of WW2, by David Brown, pub. by Arms & Armour Press, 1990.

Name Index

Name	Latitude	Longitude	Area	Page	Wreck
A W Singleton	56 09 30 N PA	03 03 30 W PA	Methil	102	133
Aberavon	55 57 45 N PA	02 23 00 W PA	Dunbar	36	25
Abertay ?	56 00 57 N	03 21 12 W	Inchcolm	90	113
Adam Smith	56 05 36 N PA	03 09 00 W PA	Kirkcaldy	100	127
Agnes	55 57 45 N PA	02 23 00 W PA	Dunbar	37	29
Alekto	56 01 26 N	03 04 20 W	May	114	157
Alfred Erlandsen	55 53 42 N	02 07 14 W	St. Abbs	25	8
Alliance ?	56 01 14 N	03 18 27 W	Inchcolm	91	114
Alloa	56 11 00 N PA	02 35 30 W PA	May	124	178
Alma	56 40 00 N PA	02 26 00 W PA	Montrose	183	285
Andreas	56 17 00 N PA	02 35 00 W PA	Fife Ness	154	224
Andromeda	55 57 45 N PA	02 23 00 W PA	Dunbar	36	27
Anlaby	56 11 15 N	02 33 52 W	May	127	184
Annette	56 17 00 N PA	02 35 00 W PA	Fife Ness	155	228
Annie Cowley	56 01 30 N PA	03 08 00 W PA	Inchkeith	76	95
Ansgar	56 11 42 N	02 47 00 W	Elie	110	153
Antelope	56 10 30 N PA	03 00 45 W PA	Methil	103	135
Anu	56 26 54 N	02 35 41 W	Tay	170	259
Arcturus			Unknown	199	320
Argyll	56 26 00 N	02 23 30 W	Arbroath	175	273
Arizona	56 10 14 N	02 52 23 W	Elie	108	148
Ashgrove	56 11 00 N	03 00 12 W	Methil	104	138
Asta	56 10 11 N	02 21 34 W	May	119	169
Auriac	55 55 00 N PA	01 50 00 W PA	St. Abbs	29	13
Avondale Park	56 09 17 N	02 30 08 W	May	116	162
Axel	56 07 18 N PA	03 07 12w PA	May	124	179
Baku Standard	56 48 30 N	02 12 48 W	Gourdon	191	302
Ballochbuie ?	56 13 46 N	02 23 36 W	May	139	207
Balmoral	56 47 48 N PA	02 18 30 W PA	Gourdon	190	300
Barge G4	56 05 15 N	02 55 10 W	Aberlady	65	83
Baron Stjernblad	55 50 00 N PA	02 04 00 W PA	Berwick	22	2
Bay Fisher	56 28 09 N	02 19 12 W	Arbroath	177	276
Bayonet	55 59 50 N	03 09 54 W	Leith	66	87
Bear	55 55 00 N PA	02 06 00 W PA	St. Abbs	28	12
Beathwood	56 42 36 N	02 24 18 W	Montrose	186	293
Bellona II	56 49 24 N	02 09 30 W	Gourdon	192	304
Ben Ardna	56 27 00 N PA	02 40 00 W PA	Tay	171	261
Ben Attow	56 09 36 N	02 26 00 W	May	117	164
Ben Heilem	55 46 01 N	01 59 00 W	Berwick	22	1
Ben Screel	55 54 00 N	02 05 00 W PA	St. Abbs	27	10
Bjornhaug	56 17 12 N	02 34 30 W	Fife Ness	156	231
Blackmorevale	56 37 24 N	02 09 06 W	Montrose	182	282
Blackwhale	56 20 00 N PA	02 30 00 W PA	Fife Ness	162	246
Boy Andrew	56 03 31 N	03 01 55 W	Inchkeith	86	109
Boyne Castle	56 07 00 N PA	02 09 00 W PA	Dunbar	45	51
Braconburn	56 25 00 N PA	02 20 00 W PA	Arbroath	174	271
Bull	56 04 30 N PA	02 43 00 W PA	N.Berwick	53	63

Shipwrecks of the Forth

Name	Latitude	Longitude	Area	Page	Wreck
Calceolaria	56 27 00 N PA	02 40 00 W PA	Tay	170	260
Campania	56 02 26 N	03 13 20 W	Inchkeith	80	104
Carl Konow	56 11 25 N PA	02 34 00 W PA	May	129	187
Carmen of Stockholm	56 11 18 N	02 33 15 W	May	128	185
Cerne	56 30 21 N	02 36 24 W	Arbroath	178	278
Charles Hammond ?	56 09 05 N	02 57 31 W	Methil	102	132
Chester II	56 04 16 N	02 52 15 W	Aberlady	64	82
Chingford	56 15 58 N	02 35 46 W	Fife Ness	151	219
Clan Shaw	56 26 28 N	02 38 43 W	Tay	169	258
Clint	56 42 12 N	02 24 30 W	Montrose	185	290
Columba	56 09 30 N	02 33 30 W	May	117	163
Commodore	56 17 00 N PA	02 35 00 W PA	Fife Ness	155	227
Cradock	56 05 00 N PA	02 00 00 W PA	Dunbar	43	47
Cramond Island	55 52 30 N	02 01 00 W	St. Abbs	25	6
Cushendall	56 57 38 N	02 04 00 W	Stonehaven	197	316
Cyclops	56 03 43 N	02 29 38 W	Dunbar	43	45
Cydum	55 57 45 N PA	02 23 00 W PA	Dunbar	37	30
Dante	56 12 00 N PA	02 46 00 W PA	Elie	110	154
Deerhound ?	56 01 12 N	03 06 38 W	Inchkeith	71	90
Desabla	56 54 54 N	01 47 18 W	Stonehaven	196	312
Dove	55 56 30 N PA	02 16 00 W PA	St. Abbs	32	19
Downiehills	56 16 46 N PA	02 34 52 W PA	Fife Ness	153	223
Duna ?	56 06 59 N	02 49 18 W	N.Berwick	57	69
Dunbritton	56 11 00 N PA	02 33 00 W PA	May	125	180
Dunscore ?	55 58 12 N	02 01 06 W	St. Abbs	34	22
Durham Coast	56 11 30 N PA	02 33 30 W PA	May	130	189
Ecclefechan	55 59 42 N	02 26 24 W	Dunbar	40	36
Echo	56 57 18 N PA	02 11 45 W PA	Stonehaven	196	313
Egholm	55 50 00 N PA	01 52 00 W PA	Berwick	23	3
Einar Jarl	56 17 30 N PA	02 18 00 W PA	Fife Ness	157	233
Elcho Castle	56 01 00 N	03 24 48 W	Rosyth	96	125
Eliza	56 03 24 N PA	02 37 30 W PA	N.Berwick	58	71
Elterwater	56 03 06 N	02 36 48 W	N.Berwick	51	58
Emley	56 10 38 N	02 33 32 W	May	120	172
Fairy Queen	56 17 12 N	02 34 30 W	Fife Ness	156	230
Fertile Vale	56 26 10 N	02 39 18 W	Tay	169	257
Festing Grindall	56 17 45 N	02 34 30 W	Fife Ness	160	239
Footah	56 12 00 N PA	02 35 00 W PA	May	136	200
Fortuna	55 52 30 N	02 00 00 W	St. Abbs	25	7
Fountains Abbey	56 37 00 N PA	02 29 00 W PA	Arbroath	179	281
Fox	56 00 30 N PA	02 30 30 W PA	Dunbar	41	39
Fri	56 00 18 N	03 25 00 W	Rosyth	93	119
Frigga	56 00 30 N PA	02 30 24 W PA	Dunbar	41	40
Frons Oliviae	56 27 00 N PA	02 40 00 W PA	Tay	171	262
Gareloch	56 12 30 N	02 44 00 W	Elie	111	155
Garibaldi	56 10 50 N PA	02 32 30 W PA	May	122	176
Gasray	55 56 00 N PA	02 09 00 W PA	St. Abbs	31	17
George Aunger	56 11 33 N PA	02 33 30 W PA	May	132	194
Ghido	56 01 30 N PA	03 08 00 W PA	Inchkeith	76	96
Girl Eva	56 27 00 N PA	02 40 00 W PA	Tay	171	263
Girl Mary	56 01 40 N	03 18 40 W	Inchcolm	92	117
Gladstone	56 20 30 N PA	02 47 00 W PA	Fife Ness	163	248
Glanmire	55 55 02 N	02 08 07 W	St. Abbs	30	15
Gloamin	56 19 30 N PA	02 40 00 W PA	Fife Ness	162	245
Good Design	56 02 56 N	03 06 20 W	Inchkeith	85	105
Goodwill	56 03 28 N PA	03 03 00 W PA	Inchkeith	86	107

Name Index

Name	Latitude	Longitude	Area	Page	Wreck
Gowrie	56 57 24 N	02 01 42 W	Stonehaven	197	315
Graf Todleben	56 10 50 N	02 50 00 W	Elie	109	150
Granero	56 54 30 N	02 11 36 W	Stonehaven	195	311
Greenawn	56 42 00 N PA	02 05 00 W PA	Montrose	184	287
Grimsel	56 01 54 N	03 07 48 W	Inchkeith	77	98
H C Grube	56 42 00 N PA	02 26 00 W PA	Montrose	184	288
Halland	56 03 00 N PA	02 17 00 W PA	Dunbar	42	43
Harley	56 18 54 N	02 09 12 W	Fife Ness	161	243
Hawnby	56 47 42 N PA	02 19 00 W PA	Gourdon	188	298
Heima	56 03 30 N PA	03 11 00 W PA	Inchkeith	86	108
Heistad	56 43 00 N PA	02 26 00 W PA	Montrose	187	294
Herrington	56 37 12 N	02 37 36 W	Arbroath	173	269
Hilda	56 11 33 N PA	02 33 30 W PA	May	131	192
Hiram	56 01 42 N	02 35 15 W	N.Berwick	50	55
Hoche	56 30 16 N	02 36 30 W	Arbroath	177	277
Hoosac	56 10 30 N PA	02 33 30 W PA	May	121	174
Hosianna	56 00 18 N	03 24 39 W	Rosyth	94	120
Integrity ?	56 02 16 N	03 11 48 W	Inchkeith	79	103
Iris	56 04 00 N PA	03 04 00 W PA	Inchkeith	87	110
Isa Fiord	56 57 18 N PA	02 11 45 W PA	Stonehaven	196	314
Island	56 11 02 N	02 32 52 W	May	126	181
Islandmagee	56 17 30 N	02 32 18 W	Fife Ness	158	235
Ivanhoe	55 59 30 N PA	03 10 00 W PA	Leith	66	86
Jane Ross	56 16 08 N	02 35 36 W	Fife Ness	153	221
Jasper	56 11 12 N PA	02 33 03 W PA	May	127	182
John	55 57 45 N PA	02 23 00 W PA	Dunbar	36	26
Juno	56 17 00 N PA	02 35 00 W PA	Fife Ness	156	229
Jupiter	56 11 00 N PA	02 48 30 W PA	Elie	109	151
K-17	56 15 21 N	02 11 41 W	May	138	208
K-4	56 15 32 N	02 11 00 W	May	140	209
Karen	56 11 04 N	02 58 45 W	Methil	104	139
Kate Thompson	56 17 50 N	02 37 24 W	Fife Ness	160	241
Katrine	56 11 25 N	02 33 30 W	May	129	188
King Jaja	55 57 45 N PA	02 23 00 W PA	Dunbar	37	28
Kitty	56 11 39 N PA	01 45 00 W PA	Dunbar	47	54
Knot	56 17 00 N	02 34 30 W	Fife Ness	154	226
LCA 672? or LCA 811?	56 02 58 N	03 00 15 W	Aberlady	63	81
LCA 845	56 05 27 N	02 53 12 W	Aberlady	65	84
Lena Melling	56 27 00 N PA	02 40 00 W PA	Tay	172	264
Leonard			Fife Ness	148	210
Lettie	56 45 18 N PA	02 25 00 W PA	Montrose	187	295
Lingbank	56 15 10 N PA	02 32 50 W PA	Fife Ness	149	214
Linnet	56 11 12 N PA	02 33 00 W PA	May	127	183
Livlig	55 58 00 N PA	02 22 00 W PA	Dunbar	38	32
Lord Beaconsfield	56 36 22 N	02 29 30 W	Arbroath	179	280
Louise	56 16 00 N PA	02 33 00 W PA	Fife Ness	152	220
Louise Henrietta	56 11 33 N PA	02 33 30 W PA	May	132	193
Lucie	56 02 00 N PA	03 08 00 W PA	Inchkeith	78	100
Ludlow	56 03 55 N	02 45 58 W	N.Berwick	53	62
Magicienne	55 56 06 N	02 19 45 W	St. Abbs	32	18
Magne	55 51 12 N	01 55 24 W	Eyemouth	23	4
Mallard	56 11 49 N	02 35 25 W	May	135	199
Mare Vivimus	56 08 00 N	02 51 00 W	Elie	105	141
Margaret Edward	56 21 00 N PA	02 35 00 W PA	Tay	166	250
Maria	56 03 24 N PA	02 37 30 W PA	N.Berwick	52	61
Marie Elizabeth	56 17 36 N PA	02 34 30 W PA	Fife Ness	159	237

SHIPWRECKS OF THE FORTH

Name	Latitude	Longitude	Area	Page	Wreck
Mars	56 11 35 N	02 33 52 W	May	135	198
Mata Garda	56 11 33 N PA	02 33 30 W PA	May	135	197
Matador	56 59 22 N	02 04 24 W	Stonehaven	197	317
Merlin	56 20 30 N	02 47 15 W	Fife Ness	163	249
Milford Earl	56 38 42 N	02 23 48 W	Montrose	182	283
Moresby	56 06 01 N	02 31 07 W	Dunbar	44	49
Munchen	56 07 18 N	02 46 21 W	N.Berwick	58	72
Musketeer	56 17 12 N	02 34 30 W	Fife Ness	157	232
Nailsea River	56 27 35 N	02 32 18 W	Arbroath	176	275
Newcastle Packet	56 11 20 N	02 33 00 W	May	129	186
No.4 Hopper	56 10 50 N PA	03 00 30 W PA	Methil	104	137
Nordhav II	56 42 17 N	02 03 48 W	Montrose	185	291
Northumbria	56 12 26 N	02 34 43 W	May	137	202
Nyon	55 55 54 N	02 12 48 W	St. Abbs	31	16
O-13			Unknown	198	318
Odense	55 54 44 N	02 09 12 W	St. Abbs	28	11
Olivier	56 17 36 N	02 34 30 W	Fife Ness	159	238
Oscar Den II	56 01 45 N PA	03 08 00 W PA	Inchkeith	77	97
Othonna	56 15 00 N PA	02 30 00 W PA	Fife Ness	149	212
Pansy	56 46 40 N PA	02 21 40 W PA	Gourdon	188	296
Paolo	56 01 24 N PA	03 10 30 W PA	Inchkeith	74	93
Pathfinder	56 07 18 N	02 09 20 W	Dunbar	46	52
Paul	56 02 00 N PA	03 08 00 W PA	Inchkeith	78	101
Phaeacian	56 09 20 N	02 52 32 W	Elie	107	145
Phineas Beard	56 38 45 N	02 26 06 W	Montrose	183	284
Pladda	56 15 45 N	02 36 00 W	Fife Ness	151	218
Plethos	56 42 00 N PA	02 05 00 W PA	Montrose	185	289
Poderosa	56 03 00 N PA	02 36 30 W PA	N.Berwick	50	57
Porthcawl	56 01 36 N	03 18 36 W	Inchcolm	92	116
President	55 52 05 N	02 04 15 W	Eyemouth	24	5
Primrose	56 10 42 N PA	02 33 21 W PA	May	121	173
Prosum	55 57 45 N PA	02 23 00 W PA	Dunbar	38	31
Protector	56 27 25 N	02 41 34 W	Tay	172	266
Queen	56 17 00 N	02 34 30 W	Fife Ness	154	225
Queensbury	56 47 48 N	02 10 48 W	Gourdon	190	299
Queensland ?	56 13 42 N	02 24 12 W	May	138	206
Quickstep	56 01 12 N PA	03 07 24 W PA	Inchkeith	90	112
Quixotic	56 26 00 N	02 23 00 W	Arbroath	176	274
Rap	56 12 30 N PA	02 57 00 W PA	Methil	105	140
Reindeer	56 52 00 N PA	02 13 00 W PA	Stonehaven	193	309
Repro	56 51 00 N	02 08 30 W	Gourdon	193	307
Ribnitz	55 58 42 N PA	02 25 00 W PA	Dunbar	39	34
River Avon	56 15 38 N	02 35 30 W	Fife Ness	150	217
River Garry	55 58 00 N PA	02 22 00 W PA	Dunbar	39	33
Rolfsborg	56 08 13 N	02 52 03 W	Elie	105	142
Royal Archer	56 06 26 N	02 59 56 W	Kirkcaldy	101	128
Royal Fusilier	56 06 32 N	02 35 18 W	N.Berwick	55	68
Ruby	56 00 34 N	03 26 50 W	Rosyth	96	124
Runswick ?	56 01 17 N	03 04 42 W	Inchkeith	72	92
Sabbia	56 06 12 N	02 25 18 W	Dunbar	45	50
Salem	56 20 05 N	02 48 00 W	Fife Ness	162	247
Salvestria	56 04 03 N	03 04 07 W	Inchkeith	88	111
Sappho ?	56 01 26 N	03 04 20 W	Inchkeith	74	94
Saucy	56 02 10 N	03 10 33 W	Inchkeith	79	102
Savant	56 15 30 N PA	02 36 00 W PA	Fife Ness	150	216
Scandia	55 59 00 N PA	02 26 00 W PA	Dunbar	39	35

Name Index

Name	Latitude	Longitude	Area	Page	Wreck
Scio	56 10 30 N PA	03 01 00 W PA	Methil	103	136
Scotland	56 10 50 N PA	02 32 30 W PA	May	124	177
Skulda	56 00 24 N	03 25 05 W	Rosyth	95	122
Sneland 1	56 09 40 N	02 30 48 W	May	118	165
Snowdrop	56 03 20 N PA	03 05 12 W PA	Inchkeith	85	106
Soar	56 49 10 N PA	02 17 20 W PA	Gourdon	191	303
Sophie	56 02 30 N PA	02 36 30 W PA	N.Berwick	50	56
Sophron	56 23 30 N	02 35 45 W	Tay	167	253
Spey	56 15 00 N PA	02 30 00 W PA	Fife Ness	149	213
Stancourt	56 25 52 N	02 44 22 W	Tay	168	256
Stella	56 05 00 N PA	02 38 00 W PA	N.Berwick	54	65
Stella Maris	56 00 00 N PA	02 29 30 W	Dunbar	40	37
Stjernvik	56 07 45 N	02 41 00 W	N.Berwick	59	74
Storjen (OB 71)	56 14 51 N	02 27 12 W	Fife Ness	148	211
Strathrannoch	55 55 00 N PA	02 07 00 W PA	St. Abbs	29	14
Success	56 18 00 N	02 37 36 W	Fife Ness	161	242
Sunbeam 1	56 02 00 N PA	03 08 00 W PA	Inchkeith	78	99
Sutlej	56 27 00 N PA	02 42 30 W PA	Tay	172	265
Switha	56 01 11 N	03 06 38 W	Inchkeith	70	89
Tanevik	56 51 48 N	01 55 42 W	Gourdon	193	308
Taurus	56 49 30 N PA	02 09 00 W PA	Gourdon	192	305
Telesilla	56 00 22 N	03 24 12 W	Rosyth	94	121
Tempo?	55 57 30 N PA	01 41 00 W PA	St. Abbs	34	21
The Broders	56 11 00 N PA	02 48 30 W PA	Elie	110	152
Thomas Alfred	56 03 24 N PA	02 37 30 W PA	N.Berwick	51	60
Thomas L Devlin	56 11 33 N	02 33 54 W	May	133	196
Thorgny	56 10 12 N PA	03 01 30 W PA	Methil	103	134
Thrive	56 10 23 N	02 20 06 W	May	120	171
Thura	56 00 03 N PA	03 23 00 W PA	Rosyth	93	118
Tillycorthie	55 53 50 N PA	01 44 00 W PA	St. Abbs	27	9
Tordenskjold	56 15 00 N PA	02 48 00 W PA	Tay	167	254
Triumph VI?	56 02 00 N	03 34 03 W	Rosyth	97	126
Tyr	56 00 27 N PA	03 22 30 W PA	Rosyth	95	123
U-12	56 07 12 N	02 20 00 W	May	114	156
U-398			Unknown	199	319
U-714	55 57 00 N PA	01 57 00 W PA	St. Abbs	34	20
UB63	56 10 00 N PA	02 00 00 W PA	May	118	167
UC-41	56 25 44 N	02 36 27 W	Tay	168	255
Ugie (possibly)	56 22 59 N	02 27 40 W	Tay	166	252
Unknown	55 58 12 N	03 01 32 W	Leith	65	85
Unknown	56 00 30 N PA	02 13 00 W PA	Dunbar	40	38
Unknown	56 01 24 N	02 57 24 W	Aberlady	62	78
Unknown	56 01 30 N PA	02 05 30 W PA	Dunbar	41	41
Unknown	56 01 52 N	02 52 20 W	Aberlady	62	79
Unknown	56 02 00 N PA	02 12 00 W PA	Dunbar	42	42
Unknown	56 04 45 N PA	02 38 30 W PA	N.Berwick	54	64
Unknown	56 05 20 N	02 24 53 W	Dunbar	44	48
Unknown	56 07 00 N	02 45 42 W	N.Berwick	57	70
Unknown	56 08 18 N	02 58 21 W	Methil	101	130
Unknown	56 08 30 N PA	02 28 18 W PA	May	115	159
Unknown	56 08 58 N	02 56 57 W	Methil	102	131
Unknown	56 10 11 N	02 32 37 W	May	120	170
Unknown	56 11 30 N PA	02 11 30 W PA	May	130	190
Unknown	56 15 27 N	02 22 54 W	Fife Ness	150	215
Unknown	56 17 36 N	02 19 30 W	Fife Ness	158	236
Unknown	56 17 48 N	02 24 06 W	Fife Ness	160	240

Name	Latitude	Longitude	Area	Page	Wreck
Unknown	56 21 46 N	02 12 12 W	Arbroath	173	267
Unknown	56 22 40 N	02 16 48 W	Arbroath	173	268
Unknown	56 22 54 N	02 48 51 W	Tay	166	251
Unknown	56 23 00 N	02 16 36 W	Arbroath	174	270
Unknown	56 25 06 N	02 14 00 W	Arbroath	175	272
Unknown	56 49 30 N	02 12 36 W	Gourdon	192	306
Unknown	56 53 04 N	02 03 12 W	Stonehaven	194	310
Unknown - 1930s ?	56 05 14 N	02 49 43 W	N.Berwick	54	66
Unknown - 3 Barges	56 01 24 N	03 21 24 W	Inchcolm	91	115
Unknown - Adoration?	56 03 10 N	02 16 50 W	Dunbar	42	44
Unknown - Ballochbuie?	56 13 41 N	02 14 00 W	May	138	205
Unknown - Barge	56 00 42 N	02 56 20 W	Aberlady	60	76
Unknown - Ben Attow?	56 12 49 N	02 24 58 W	May	138	204
Unknown - Canganian?	56 35 24 N	02 21 30 W	Arbroath	178	279
Unknown - Eber ?	56 09 42 N	02 21 15 W	May	118	166
Unknown - Greenawn ?	56 42 18 N	02 07 30 W	Montrose	186	292
Unknown - LH308 ?	56 41 39 N	02 07 30 W	Montrose	184	286
Unknown - Mallard?	56 11 30 N PA	02 28 30 W PA	May	131	191
Unknown - Pre 1919	56 08 18 N	02 32 40 W	May	115	158
Unknown - Pre 1919	56 10 10 N	02 18 45 W	May	119	168
Unknown - Pre 1919	56 12 20 N PA	02 33 10 W PA	May	136	201
Unknown - Pre 1935	56 07 31 N	02 49 04 W	N.Berwick	58	73
Unknown - Pre 1939	56 09 17 N	02 52 51 W	Elie	106	144
Unknown - Pre 1940	56 08 22 N	02 48 51 W	Elie	106	143
Unknown - Pre 1940	56 09 39 N	02 53 19 W	Elie	107	146
Unknown - Pre 1940	56 47 50 N	02 09 36 W	Gourdon	191	301
Unknown - Pre 1946	56 07 23 N	03 05 23 W	Kirkcaldy	101	129
Unknown - Pre 1952	56 00 10 N	03 09 40 W	Leith	67	88
Unknown - Pre 1959	56 02 15 N	02 54 33 W	Aberlady	63	80
Unknown - Pre 1962	56 08 17 N	02 44 46 W	N.Berwick	59	75
Unknown - Pre 1979	56 06 06 N	02 50 06 W	N.Berwick	55	67
Unknown - Rockingham ?	56 19 00 N	02 17 12 W	Fife Ness	161	244
Unknown - U-Boat ?	56 09 45 N	02 50 45 W	Elie	107	147
Unknown - U-Boat ?	56 47 12 N	02 11 48 W	Gourdon	188	297
Unknown - UB-63 ?	56 10 30 N PA	02 24 00 W PA	May	122	175
Unknown - UB-63 ?	56 08 57 N	01 54 30 W	May	115	160
Unknown - WW2	56 09 00 N PA	02 38 00 W PA	May	115	161
Unknown - WW2 ?	56 04 00 N PA	02 21 00 W PA	Dunbar	43	46
Unknown - WW2 ?	56 12 30 N PA	02 27 00 W PA	May	137	203
Unknown X-Craft	56 01 21 N	02 52 45 W	Aberlady	60	77
Unknown X-Craft	56 01 26 N	02 53 09 W	Aberlady	60	77
Utopia	56 00 00 N PA	01 49 30 W PA	St. Abbs	35	24
Valhalla	56 03 20 N PA	02 38 45 W PA	N.Berwick	51	59
Verbormilia	56 00 00 N PA	02 14 00 W PA	St. Abbs	35	23
Victory	56 11 33 N PA	02 33 30 W PA	May	132	195
Vigilant	56 01 15 N PA	03 07 18 W PA	Inchkeith	72	91
Vildfugl	56 16 45 N	02 35 00 W	Fife Ness	153	222
Vulcan	56 10 45 N PA	02 50 30 W PA	Elie	108	149
Windsor Castle	56 17 30 N PA	02 35 00 W PA	Fife Ness	157	234
ZZ12	56 09 00 N	02 13 07 W	Dunbar	46	53

Latitude Index

Latitude	Longitude	Name	Area	Page	Wreck
55 46 01 N	01 59 00 W	Ben Heilem	Berwick	22	1
55 50 00 N PA	01 52 00 W PA	Egholm	Berwick	23	3
55 50 00 N PA	02 04 00 W PA	Baron Stjernblad	Berwick	22	2
55 51 12 N	01 55 24 W	Magne	Eyemouth	23	4
55 52 05 N	02 04 15 W	President	Eyemouth	24	5
55 52 30 N	02 00 00 W	Fortuna	St. Abbs	25	7
55 52 30 N	02 01 00 W	Cramond Island	St. Abbs	25	6
55 53 42 N	02 07 14 W	Alfred Erlandsen	St. Abbs	25	8
55 53 50 N PA	01 44 00 W PA	Tillycorthie	St. Abbs	27	9
55 54 00 N PA	02 05 00 W PA	Ben Screel	St. Abbs	27	10
55 54 44 N	02 09 12 W	Odense	St. Abbs	28	11
55 55 00 N PA	01 50 00 W PA	Auriac	St. Abbs	29	13
55 55 00 N PA	02 06 00 W PA	Bear	St. Abbs	28	12
55 55 00 N PA	02 07 00 W PA	Strathrannoch	St. Abbs	29	14
55 55 02 N	02 08 07 W	Glanmire	St. Abbs	30	15
55 55 54 N	02 12 48 W	Nyon	St. Abbs	31	16
55 56 00 N PA	02 09 00 W PA	Gasray	St. Abbs	31	17
55 56 06 N	02 19 45 W	Magicienne	St. Abbs	32	18
55 56 30 N PA	02 16 00 W PA	Dove	St. Abbs	32	19
55 57 00 N PA	01 57 00 W PA	U-714	St. Abbs	34	20
55 57 30 N PA	01 41 00 W PA	Tempo?	St. Abbs	34	21
55 57 45 N PA	02 23 00 W PA	Aberavon	Dunbar	36	25
55 57 45 N PA	02 23 00 W PA	Agnes	Dunbar	37	29
55 57 45 N PA	02 23 00 W PA	Andromeda	Dunbar	36	27
55 57 45 N PA	02 23 00 W PA	Cydum	Dunbar	37	30
55 57 45 N PA	02 23 00 W PA	John	Dunbar	36	26
55 57 45 N PA	02 23 00 W PA	King Jaja	Dunbar	37	28
55 57 45 N PA	02 23 00 W PA	Prosum	Dunbar	38	31
55 58 00 N PA	02 22 00 W PA	Livlig	Dunbar	38	32
55 58 00 N PA	02 22 00 W PA	River Garry	Dunbar	39	33
55 58 12 N	02 01 06 W	Dunscore ?	St. Abbs	34	22
55 58 12 N	03 01 32 W	Unknown	Leith	65	85
55 58 42 N PA	02 25 00 W PA	Ribnitz	Dunbar	39	34
55 59 00 N PA	02 26 00 W PA	Scandia	Dunbar	39	35
55 59 30 N PA	03 10 00 W PA	Ivanhoe	Leith	66	86
55 59 42 N	02 26 24 W	Ecclefechan	Dunbar	40	36
55 59 50 N	03 09 54 W	Bayonet	Leith	66	87
56 00 00 N PA	01 49 30 W PA	Utopia	St. Abbs	35	24
56 00 00 N PA	02 14 00 W PA	Verbormilia	St. Abbs	35	23
56 00 00 N PA	02 29 30 W	Stella Maris	Dunbar	40	37
56 00 03 N PA	03 23 00 W PA	Thura	Rosyth	93	118
56 00 10 N	03 09 40 W	Unknown - Pre 1952	Leith	67	88
56 00 18 N	03 24 39 W	Hosianna	Rosyth	94	120
56 00 18 N	03 25 00 W	Fri	Rosyth	93	119
56 00 22 N	03 24 12 W	Telesilla	Rosyth	94	121
56 00 24 N	03 25 05 W	Skulda	Rosyth	95	122

Shipwrecks of the Forth

Latitude	Longitude	Name	Area	Page	Wreck
56 00 27 N PA	03 22 30 W PA	Tyr	Rosyth	95	123
56 00 30 N PA	02 13 00 W PA	Unknown	Dunbar	40	38
56 00 30 N PA	02 30 24 W PA	Frigga	Dunbar	41	40
56 00 30 N PA	02 30 30 W PA	Fox	Dunbar	41	39
56 00 34 N	03 26 50 W	Ruby	Rosyth	96	124
56 00 42 N	02 56 20 W	Unknown - Barge	Aberlady	60	76
56 00 57 N	03 21 12 W	Abertay ?	Inchcolm	90	113
56 01 00 N	03 24 48 W	Elcho Castle	Rosyth	96	125
56 01 11 N	03 06 38 W	Switha	Inchkeith	70	89
56 01 12 N	03 06 38 W	Deerhound ?	Inchkeith	71	90
56 01 12 N PA	03 07 24 W PA	Quickstep	Inchkeith	90	112
56 01 14 N	03 18 27 W	Alliance ?	Inchcolm	91	114
56 01 15 N PA	03 07 18 W PA	Vigilant	Inchkeith	72	91
56 01 17 N	03 04 42 W	Runswick ?	Inchkeith	72	92
56 01 21 N	02 52 45 W	Unknown X-Craft	Aberlady	60	77
56 01 24 N	02 57 24 W	Unknown	Aberlady	62	78
56 01 24 N	03 21 24 W	Unknown - 3 Barges	Inchcolm	91	115
56 01 24 N PA	03 10 30 W PA	Paolo	Inchkeith	74	93
56 01 26 N	02 53 09 W	Unknown X-Craft	Aberlady	60	77
56 01 26 N	03 04 20 W	Sappho ?	Inchkeith	74	94
56 01 26 N	03 04 20 W	Alekto	May	114	157
56 01 30 N PA	02 05 30 W PA	Unknown	Dunbar	41	41
56 01 30 N PA	03 08 00 W PA	Annie Cowley	Inchkeith	76	95
56 01 30 N PA	03 08 00 W PA	Ghido	Inchkeith	76	96
56 01 36 N	03 18 36 W	Porthcawl	Inchcolm	92	116
56 01 40 N	03 18 40 W	Girl Mary	Inchcolm	92	117
56 01 42 N	02 35 15 W	Hiram	N.Berwick	50	55
56 01 45 N PA	03 08 00 W PA	Oscar Den II	Inchkeith	77	97
56 01 52 N	02 52 20 W	Unknown	Aberlady	62	79
56 01 54 N	03 07 48 W	Grimsel	Inchkeith	77	98
56 02 00 N	03 34 03 W	Triumph VI?	Rosyth	97	126
56 02 00 N PA	02 12 00 W PA	Unknown	Dunbar	42	42
56 02 00 N PA	03 08 00 W PA	Lucie	Inchkeith	78	100
56 02 00 N PA	03 08 00 W PA	Paul	Inchkeith	78	101
56 02 00 N PA	03 08 00 W PA	Sunbeam 1	Inchkeith	78	99
56 02 10 N	03 10 33 W	Saucy	Inchkeith	79	102
56 02 15 N	02 54 33 W	Unknown - Pre 1959	Aberlady	63	80
56 02 16 N	03 11 48 W	Integrity ?	Inchkeith	79	103
56 02 26 N	03 13 20 W	Campania	Inchkeith	80	104
56 02 30 N PA	02 36 30 W PA	Sophie	N.Berwick	50	56
56 02 56 N	03 06 20 W	Good Design	Inchkeith	85	105
56 02 58 N	03 00 15 W	LCA 672? or LCA 811?	Aberlady	63	81
56 03 00 N PA	02 17 00 W PA	Halland	Dunbar	42	43
56 03 00 N PA	02 36 30 W PA	Poderosa	N.Berwick	50	57
56 03 06 N	02 36 48 W	Elterwater	N.Berwick	51	58
56 03 10 N	02 16 50 W	Unknown - Adoration?	Dunbar	42	44
56 03 20 N PA	02 38 45 W PA	Valhalla	N.Berwick	51	59
56 03 20 N PA	03 05 12 W PA	Snowdrop	Inchkeith	85	106
56 03 24 N PA	02 37 30 W PA	Eliza	N.Berwick	58	71
56 03 24 N PA	02 37 30 W PA	Maria	N.Berwick	52	61
56 03 24 N PA	02 37 30 W PA	Thomas Alfred	N.Berwick	51	60
56 03 28 N PA	03 03 00 W PA	Goodwill	Inchkeith	86	107
56 03 30 N PA	03 11 00 W PA	Heima	Inchkeith	86	108
56 03 31 N	03 01 55 W	Boy Andrew	Inchkeith	86	109
56 03 43 N	02 29 38 W	Cyclops	Dunbar	43	45
56 03 55 N	02 45 58 W	Ludlow	N.Berwick	53	62

210

Latitude Index

Latitude	Longitude	Name	Area	Page	Wreck
56 04 00 N PA	02 21 00 W PA	Unknown - WW2 ?	Dunbar	43	46
56 04 00 N PA	03 04 00 W PA	Iris	Inchkeith	87	110
56 04 03 N	03 04 07 W	Salvestria	Inchkeith	88	111
56 04 16 N	02 52 15 W	Chester II	Aberlady	64	82
56 04 30 N PA	02 43 00 W PA	Bull	N.Berwick	53	63
56 04 45 N PA	02 38 30 W PA	Unknown	N.Berwick	54	64
56 05 00 N PA	02 00 00 W PA	Cradock	Dunbar	43	47
56 05 00 N PA	02 38 00 W PA	Stella	N.Berwick	54	65
56 05 14 N	02 49 43 W	Unknown - 1930s ?	N.Berwick	54	66
56 05 15 N	02 55 10 W	Barge G4	Aberlady	65	83
56 05 20 N	02 24 53 W	Unknown	Dunbar	44	48
56 05 27 N	02 53 12 W	LCA 845	Aberlady	65	84
56 05 36 N PA	03 09 00 W PA	Adam Smith	Kirkcaldy	100	127
56 06 01 N	02 31 07 W	Moresby	Dunbar	44	49
56 06 06 N	02 50 06 W	Unknown - Pre 1979	N.Berwick	55	67
56 06 12 N	02 25 18 W	Sabbia	Dunbar	45	50
56 06 26 N	02 59 56 W	Royal Archer	Kirkcaldy	101	128
56 06 32 N	02 35 18 W	Royal Fusilier	N.Berwick	55	68
56 06 59 N	02 49 18 W	Duna ?	N.Berwick	57	69
56 07 00 N	02 45 42 W	Unknown	N.Berwick	57	70
56 07 00 N PA	02 09 00 W PA	Boyne Castle	Dunbar	45	51
56 07 12 N	02 20 00 W	U-12	May	114	156
56 07 18 N	02 09 20 W	Pathfinder	Dunbar	46	52
56 07 18 N	02 46 21 W	Munchen	N.Berwick	58	72
56 07 18 N PA	03 07 12w PA	Axel	May	124	179
56 07 23 N	03 05 23 W	Unknown - Pre 1946	Kirkcaldy	101	129
56 07 31 N	02 49 04 W	Unknown - Pre 1935	N.Berwick	58	73
56 07 45 N	02 41 00 W	Stjernvik	N.Berwick	59	74
56 08 00 N	02 51 00 W	Mare Vivimus	Elie	105	141
56 08 13 N	02 52 03 W	Rolfsborg	Elie	105	142
56 08 17 N	02 44 46 W	Unknown - Pre 1962	N.Berwick	59	75
56 08 18 N	02 32 40 W	Unknown - Pre 1919	May	115	158
56 08 18 N	02 58 21 W	Unknown	Methil	101	130
56 08 22 N	02 48 51 W	Unknown - Pre 1940	Elie	106	143
56 08 30 N PA	02 28 18 W PA	Unknown	May	115	159
56 08 57 N	01 54 30 W	Unknown - UB-63 ?	May	115	160
56 08 58 N	02 56 57 W	Unknown	Methil	102	131
56 09 00 N	02 13 07 W	ZZ12	Dunbar	46	53
56 09 00 N PA	02 38 00 W PA	Unknown - WW2	May	115	161
56 09 05 N	02 57 31 W	Charles Hammond ?	Methil	102	132
56 09 17 N	02 30 08 W	Avondale Park	May	116	162
56 09 17 N	02 52 51 W	Unknown - Pre 1939	Elie	106	144
56 09 20 N	02 52 32 W	Phaeacian	Elie	107	145
56 09 30 N	02 33 30 W	Columba	May	117	163
56 09 30 N PA	03 03 30 W PA	A W Singleton	Methil	102	133
56 09 36 N	02 26 00 W	Ben Attow	May	117	164
56 09 39 N	02 53 19 W	Unknown - Pre 1940	Elie	107	146
56 09 40 N	02 30 48 W	Sneland 1	May	118	165
56 09 42 N	02 21 15 W	Unknown - Eber ?	May	118	166
56 09 45 N	02 50 45 W	Unknown - U-Boat ?	Elie	107	147
56 10 00 N PA	02 00 00 W PA	UB63	May	118	167
56 10 10 N	02 18 45 W	Unknown - Pre 1919	May	119	168
56 10 11 N	02 21 34 W	Asta	May	119	169
56 10 11 N	02 32 37 W	Unknown	May	120	170
56 10 12 N PA	03 01 30 W PA	Thorgny	Methil	103	134
56 10 14 N	02 52 23 W	Arizona	Elie	108	148

211

Shipwrecks of the Forth

Latitude	Longitude	Name	Area	Page	Wreck
56 10 23 N	02 20 06 W	Thrive	May	120	171
56 10 30 N PA	02 24 00 W PA	Unknown - UB-63 ?	May	122	175
56 10 30 N PA	02 33 30 W PA	Hoosac	May	121	174
56 10 30 N PA	03 00 45 W PA	Antelope	Methil	103	135
56 10 30 N PA	03 01 00 W PA	Scio	Methil	103	136
56 10 38 N	02 33 32 W	Emley	May	120	172
56 10 42 N PA	02 33 21 W PA	Primrose	May	121	173
56 10 45 N PA	02 50 30 W PA	Vulcan	Elie	108	149
56 10 50 N	02 50 00 W	Graf Todleben	Elie	109	150
56 10 50 N PA	02 32 30 W PA	Garibaldi	May	122	176
56 10 50 N PA	02 32 30 W PA	Scotland	May	124	177
56 10 50 N PA	03 00 30 W PA	No.4 Hopper	Methil	104	137
56 11 00 N	03 00 12 W	Ashgrove	Methil	104	138
56 11 00 N PA	02 33 00 W PA	Dunbritton	May	125	180
56 11 00 N PA	02 35 30 W PA	Alloa	May	124	178
56 11 00 N PA	02 48 30 W PA	Jupiter	Elie	109	151
56 11 00 N PA	02 48 30 W PA	The Broders	Elie	110	152
56 11 02 N	02 32 52 W	Island	May	126	181
56 11 04 N	02 58 45 W	Karen	Methil	104	139
56 11 12 N PA	02 33 00 W PA	Linnet	May	127	183
56 11 12 N PA	02 33 03 W PA	Jasper	May	127	182
56 11 15 N	02 33 52 W	Anlaby	May	127	184
56 11 18 N	02 33 15 W	Carmen of Stockholm	May	128	185
56 11 20 N	02 33 00 W	Newcastle Packet	May	129	186
56 11 25 N	02 33 30 W	Katrine	May	129	188
56 11 25 N PA	02 34 00 W PA	Carl Konow	May	129	187
56 11 30 N PA	02 11 30 W PA	Unknown	May	130	190
56 11 30 N PA	02 28 30 W PA	Unknown - Mallard?	May	131	191
56 11 30 N PA	02 33 30 W PA	Durham Coast	May	130	189
56 11 33 N	02 33 54 W	Thomas L Devlin	May	133	196
56 11 33 N PA	02 33 30 W PA	George Aunger	May	132	194
56 11 33 N PA	02 33 30 W PA	Hilda	May	131	192
56 11 33 N PA	02 33 30 W PA	Louise Henrietta	May	132	193
56 11 33 N PA	02 33 30 W PA	Mata Garda	May	135	197
56 11 33 N PA	02 33 30 W PA	Victory	May	132	195
56 11 35 N	02 33 52 W	Mars	May	135	198
56 11 39 N PA	01 45 00 W PA	Kitty	Dunbar	47	54
56 11 42 N	02 47 00 W	Ansgar	Elie	110	153
56 11 49 N	02 35 25 W	Mallard	May	135	199
56 12 00 N PA	02 35 00 W PA	Footah	May	136	200
56 12 00 N PA	02 46 00 W PA	Dante	Elie	110	154
56 12 20 N PA	02 33 10 W PA	Unknown - Pre 1919	May	136	201
56 12 26 N	02 34 43 W	Northumbria	May	137	202
56 12 30 N	02 44 00 W	Gareloch	Elie	111	155
56 12 30 N PA	02 27 00 W PA	Unknown - WW2 ?	May	137	203
56 12 30 N PA	02 57 00 W PA	Rap	Methil	105	140
56 12 49 N	02 24 58 W	Unknown - Ben Attow?	May	138	204
56 13 41 N	02 14 00 W	Unknown - Ballochbuie?	May	138	205
56 13 42 N	02 24 12 W	Queensland ?	May	138	206
56 13 46 N	02 23 36 W	Ballochbuie ?	May	139	207
56 14 51 N	02 27 12 W	Storjen(OB 71)	Fife Ness	148	211
56 15 00 N PA	02 30 00 W PA	Othonna	Fife Ness	149	212
56 15 00 N PA	02 30 00 W PA	Spey	Fife Ness	149	213
56 15 00 N PA	02 48 00 W PA	Tordenskjold	Tay	167	254
56 15 10 N PA	02 32 50 W PA	Lingbank	Fife Ness	149	214
56 15 21 N	02 11 41 W	K-17	May	138	208

Latitude Index

Latitude	Longitude	Name	Area	Page	Wreck
56 15 27 N	02 22 54 W	Unknown	Fife Ness	150	215
56 15 30 N PA	02 36 00 W PA	Savant	Fife Ness	150	216
56 15 32 N	02 11 00 W	K-4	May	140	209
56 15 38 N	02 35 30 W	River Avon	Fife Ness	150	217
56 15 45 N	02 36 00 W	Pladda	Fife Ness	151	218
56 15 58 N	02 35 46 W	Chingford	Fife Ness	151	219
56 16 00 N PA	02 33 00 W PA	Louise	Fife Ness	152	220
56 16 08 N	02 35 36 W	Jane Ross	Fife Ness	153	221
56 16 45 N	02 35 00 W	Vildfugl	Fife Ness	153	222
56 16 46 N PA	02 34 52 W PA	Downiehills	Fife Ness	153	223
56 17 00 N	02 34 30 W	Knot	Fife Ness	154	226
56 17 00 N	02 34 30 W	Queen	Fife Ness	154	225
56 17 00 N PA	02 35 00 W PA	Andreas	Fife Ness	154	224
56 17 00 N PA	02 35 00 W PA	Annette	Fife Ness	155	228
56 17 00 N PA	02 35 00 W PA	Commodore	Fife Ness	155	227
56 17 00 N PA	02 35 00 W PA	Juno	Fife Ness	156	229
56 17 12 N	02 34 30 W	Bjornhaug	Fife Ness	156	231
56 17 12 N	02 34 30 W	Fairy Queen	Fife Ness	156	230
56 17 12 N	02 34 30 W	Musketeer	Fife Ness	157	232
56 17 30 N	02 32 18 W	Islandmagee	Fife Ness	158	235
56 17 30 N PA	02 18 00 W PA	Einar Jarl	Fife Ness	157	233
56 17 30 N PA	02 35 00 W PA	Windsor Castle	Fife Ness	157	234
56 17 36 N	02 19 30 W	Unknown	Fife Ness	158	236
56 17 36 N	02 34 30 W	Olivier	Fife Ness	159	238
56 17 36 N PA	02 34 30 W PA	Marie Elizabeth	Fife Ness	159	237
56 17 45 N	02 34 30 W	Festing Grindall	Fife Ness	160	239
56 17 48 N	02 24 06 W	Unknown	Fife Ness	160	240
56 17 50 N	02 37 24 W	Kate Thompson	Fife Ness	160	241
56 18 00 N	02 37 36 W	Success	Fife Ness	161	242
56 18 54 N	02 09 12 W	Harley	Fife Ness	161	243
56 19 00 N	02 17 12 W	Unknown - Rockingham ?	Fife Ness	161	244
56 19 30 N PA	02 40 00 W PA	Gloamin	Fife Ness	162	245
56 20 00 N PA	02 30 00 W PA	Blackwhale	Fife Ness	162	246
56 20 05 N	02 48 00 W	Salem	Fife Ness	162	247
56 20 30 N	02 47 15 W	Merlin	Fife Ness	163	249
56 20 30 N PA	02 47 00 W PA	Gladstone	Fife Ness	163	248
56 21 00 N PA	02 35 00 W PA	Margaret Edward	Tay	166	250
56 21 46 N	02 12 12 W	Unknown	Arbroath	173	267
56 22 40 N	02 16 48 W	Unknown	Arbroath	173	268
56 22 54 N	02 48 51 W	Unknown	Tay	166	251
56 22 59 N	02 27 40 W	Ugie (possibly)	Tay	166	252
56 23 00 N	02 16 36 W	Unknown	Arbroath	174	270
56 23 30 N	02 35 45 W	Sophron	Tay	167	253
56 25 00 N PA	02 20 00 W PA	Braconburn	Arbroath	174	271
56 25 06 N	02 14 00 W	Unknown	Arbroath	175	272
56 25 44 N	02 36 27 W	UC-41	Tay	168	255
56 25 52 N	02 44 22 W	Stancourt	Tay	168	256
56 26 00 N	02 23 00 W	Quixotic	Arbroath	176	274
56 26 00 N	02 23 30 W	Argyll	Arbroath	175	273
56 26 10 N	02 39 18 W	Fertile Vale	Tay	169	257
56 26 28 N	02 38 43 W	Clan Shaw	Tay	169	258
56 26 54 N	02 35 41 W	Anu	Tay	170	259
56 27 00 N PA	02 40 00 W PA	Ben Ardna	Tay	171	261
56 27 00 N PA	02 40 00 W PA	Calceolaria	Tay	170	260
56 27 00 N PA	02 40 00 W PA	Frons Oliviae	Tay	171	262
56 27 00 N PA	02 40 00 W PA	Girl Eva	Tay	171	263

Shipwrecks of the Forth

Latitude	Longitude	Name	Area	Page	Wreck
56 27 00 N PA	02 40 00 W PA	Lena Melling	Tay	172	264
56 27 00 N PA	02 42 30 W PA	Sutlej	Tay	172	265
56 27 25 N	02 41 34 W	Protector	Tay	172	266
56 27 35 N	02 32 18 W	Nailsea River	Arbroath	176	275
56 28 09 N	02 19 12 W	Bay Fisher	Arbroath	177	276
56 30 16 N	02 36 30 W	Hoche	Arbroath	177	277
56 30 21 N	02 36 24 W	Cerne	Arbroath	178	278
56 35 24 N	02 21 30 W	Unknown - Canganian?	Arbroath	178	279
56 36 22 N	02 29 30 W	Lord Beaconsfield	Arbroath	179	280
56 37 00 N PA	02 29 00 W PA	Fountains Abbey	Arbroath	179	281
56 37 12 N	02 37 36 W	Herrington	Arbroath	173	269
56 37 24 N	02 09 06 W	Blackmorevale	Montrose	182	282
56 38 42 N	02 23 48 W	Milford Earl	Montrose	182	283
56 38 45 N	02 26 06 W	Phineas Beard	Montrose	183	284
56 40 00 N PA	02 26 00 W PA	Alma	Montrose	183	285
56 41 39 N	02 07 30 W	Unknown - LH308 ?	Montrose	184	286
56 42 00 N PA	02 05 00 W PA	Greenawn	Montrose	184	287
56 42 00 N PA	02 05 00 W PA	Plethos	Montrose	185	289
56 42 00 N PA	02 26 00 W PA	H C Grube	Montrose	184	288
56 42 12 N	02 24 30 W	Clint	Montrose	185	290
56 42 17 N	02 03 48 W	Nordhav II	Montrose	185	291
56 42 18 N	02 07 30 W	Unknown - Greenawn ?	Montrose	186	292
56 42 36 N	02 24 18 W	Beathwood	Montrose	186	293
56 43 00 N PA	02 26 00 W PA	Heistad	Montrose	187	294
56 45 18 N PA	02 25 00 W PA	Lettie	Montrose	187	295
56 46 40 N PA	02 21 40 W PA	Pansy	Gourdon	188	296
56 47 12 N	02 11 48 W	Unknown - U-Boat ?	Gourdon	188	297
56 47 42 N PA	02 19 00 W PA	Hawnby	Gourdon	188	298
56 47 48 N	02 10 48 W	Queensbury	Gourdon	190	299
56 47 48 N PA	02 18 30 W PA	Balmoral	Gourdon	190	300
56 47 50 N	02 09 36 W	Unknown - Pre 1940	Gourdon	191	301
56 48 30 N	02 12 48 W	Baku Standard	Gourdon	191	302
56 49 10 N PA	02 17 20 W PA	Soar	Gourdon	191	303
56 49 24 N	02 09 30 W	Bellona II	Gourdon	192	304
56 49 30 N	02 12 36 W	Unknown	Gourdon	192	306
56 49 30 N PA	02 09 00 W PA	Taurus	Gourdon	192	305
56 51 00 N	02 08 30 W	Repro	Gourdon	193	307
56 51 48 N	01 55 42 W	Tanevik	Gourdon	193	308
56 52 00 N PA	02 13 00 W PA	Reindeer	Stonehaven	193	309
56 53 04 N	02 03 12 W	Unknown	Stonehaven	194	310
56 54 30 N	02 11 36 W	Granero	Stonehaven	195	311
56 54 54 N	01 47 18 W	Desabla	Stonehaven	196	312
56 57 18 N PA	02 11 45 W PA	Echo	Stonehaven	196	313
56 57 18 N PA	02 11 45 W PA	Isa Fiord	Stonehaven	196	314
56 57 24 N	02 01 42 W	Gowrie	Stonehaven	197	315
56 57 38 N	02 04 00 W	Cushendall	Stonehaven	197	316
56 59 22 N	02 04 24 W	Matador	Stonehaven	197	317
		Arcturus	Unknown	199	320
		Leonard	Fife Ness	148	210

Nekton Books

Diving Guides to Scotland

Nekton Books was set up in 1991 with the main purpose of publishing a comprehensive series of diving guides to the whole of Scotland.

These guides will build upon the existing *Diver* guides to Scotland written by Gordon Ridley in the early and mid 1980s. Three of these have been published by Underwater World Publications :

Dive West Scotland, 1984, 192pp
Dive North-West Scotland, 1985, 200pp
Dive Scotland: The Northern Isles & East Coast, 1992, 224pp

One further book (covering the Outer Hebrides, the Hebridean Outliers and freshwater sites) is still to be published.

The new Nekton Books booklets will each cover one specific diving area in much greater detail than was possible in the above guides. The proposed list of titles is shown overleaf.

Each booklet will extend to some 64 or more pages (of A5 size), allowing an increase by a factor of four or five over the original guides. The extra space will allow the inclusion of more and fuller dive site details, wreck stories, diagrams, photographs etc. The approach to the content of the booklets will be a development of that used in the St. Kilda guide :

Ridley, G. (1983) *St Kilda : A Submarine Guide*, 48pp

although the production and printing will be at a professional level.

A second series of books describing the shipwrecks of different areas of Scotland is also planned. This book is the first of that series.

If you would like to be placed on our mailing list please contact:

Nekton Books,
94 Brownside Road, Cambuslang, Glasgow, G72 8AG
Telephone : 041 641 4200

We would also be very pleased to receive comments and suggestions. Extra information about any of the dive sites is also most welcome.

Nekton Books titles

1. Solway Firth
2. Rhinns of Galloway
3. Ayrshire
4. Upper Clyde
5. Arran
6. Clyde Lochs
7. Kintyre & Knapdale
8. Islay
9. Jura & Slate Isles
10. Oban area
11. Loch Linnhe area
12. Sound of Mull
13. Mull
14. Coll & Tiree
15. Loch Sunart & Ardnamurchan
16. Arisaig area
17. Lochs Hourn & Nevis
18. Small Isles
19. Skye
20. Kylerhea to Applecross
21. Torridon to Gruinard Bay
22. Loch Broom & Summer Isles
23. Enard & Eddrachillis Bays
24. Handa to Faraid Head
25. North Coast & Pentland Firth
26. Moray Firth
27. Grampian
28. Firth of Forth
29. Eyemouth & Abbs
30. Freshwater
31. Orkney
32. Scapa Flow
33. Fair Isle & Foula
34. Shetland
35. Uists & Barra
36. Harris
37. Lewis
38. North Rona
39. Other Outliers
40. St. Kilda

41. Scotland for divers
42. Diving in Scotland
43. Scottish Marine Life

44. Submarines wrecked in Scottish waters
45. Warships wrecked in Scottish waters

46. Merchant shipping lost in Scottish waters 1850-1918

Please place me on your mailing list / send me further information:

Name:

Address:

My particular interests are:

I have more information on these areas:

Telephone:

Send these details to Nekton Books, 94 Brownside Road, Cambuslang, Glasgow, G72 8AG.